THE
TAO
OF
BALANCED
DIET

SECRETS OF A
THIN & HEALTHY
BODY

BY DR. STEPHEN T. CHANG

TAO PUBLISHING

Published by Tao Publishing
2700 Ocean Avenue
San Francisco, California 94132

Previously *Secrets of A Thin Body* © 1979

FIRST PRINTING 1987
SECOND PRINTING 1988
THIRD PRINTING 1992

Printed in the United States of America

Typesetting by H.S. Dakin Co., San Francisco

Library of Congress Cataloging in Publication Data

Chang, Stephen Thomas, Date
    The Tao of balanced diet.

    Includes index.
    1. Reducing diets.   2. Health.   3. Taoism.   4. Ch'i.
5. Reducing diets—Recipes.   I. Title.
RM222.2.C438 1987   613'.2'5   86-897
ISBN 0-942196-05-8

About the Author

Stephen Thomas Chang is an internationally well-known scholar. His grandmother was a master-physician, while her father was both personal physician to Empress Tse-Shi and the first Chinese ambassador to the United Kingdom. Dr. Chang has been trained in both Chinese and Western medicine, and in addition to his medical doctor degree, he holds doctor degrees in law, philosophy, and theology. He lectures world-wide on various aspects of Taoism, and he is the founder of the Foundation of Tao. He is also the author of:

The Complete Book of Acupuncture,
The Complete System of Self-Healing: Internal Exercises,
The Great Tao,
The Best Way to Make Love Work (The Tao of Sexology),
and
The Integral Management of Tao: Complete Achievement.

Several books have been translated into ten languages.

Acknowledgements

The author gratefully acknowledges the support and help of:

Helene Chang
Stephenson Chang
John Lindseth
Eugene Schwartz
Mick Winters
and Foundation of Tao

Table of Contents

Preface

Since its publication in 1979, *Secrets of a Thin Body* (the abridged edition of this book) has been generating interest in the Theory of Balanced Diet all over the world, as the first and singular informational source on the subject. In Europe alone, particularly in France, it has been received with incredible enthusiasm. From everywhere, thousands and thousands of letters have been coming in, all bearing extremely important and valuable responses. Therefore, I must take this opportunity to thank everyone deeply from my heart, to credit everyone for the depth of knowledge expressed.

In the following paragraphs I will share with you those responses, the natures of which can be categorized as follows:

1. Statements of gratitude for the diet-balancing method—Five Tastes Theory. A recapitulation of these compiled statements follows: Almost every month the world over, a new theory of dieting comes out, but almost none emphasizes dietary balance. In case dietary balance is given some consideration, few theories give complete methods for actualizing it. The wish for dietary balance has always been unrealized; no one really knows how to balance the diet, because the food territory is too large. Trying to balance the diet brings only fear, confusion, and frustration. With the introduction of the Five Tastes Theory, balancing the diet is no longer an impossible dream. With the thoroughly practicable yet simple Five Tastes theory, balancing the diet becomes extremely easy and enjoyable. The theory establishes within the mind an immediately recallable

and applicable framework for judging one's food. So as soon as the food comes within eyesight, one is able to determine whether or not it is balanced and healthy. Before the introduction of the theory, a meal holds little significance except whether or not it is delicious. After being equipped with a powerful tool to judge food, the first thought that enters the mind upon eating is not whether or not the meal tastes good but whether or not the meal is balanced (whether or not the meal is healthy). For example, when the major portion of the meal is found to be on the sour side, an objection is raised in the mind, and even though the meal may be delicious, overeating will not take place. In other words the entire perception of food has changed. Since the satisfaction derived from food is dimmed by the thought of imbalance, weight control already begins before anything is eaten or done. But when a meal is found to be balanced, the satisfaction is so great and immediate that over-eating is still prevented. Balancing one's diet with the theory results not only in improved nutrition and health, but also in weight control.

2. Comments about the recipes given in the book. The compiled comments are summarily repeated here: The meals given in the book are more than just meals; they are treats. Making a meal for oneself according to the principles listed in the book is like giving oneself a treat. When a meal is cooked for one's guests , extreme gratification shows in their faces. A balanced meal is more gratifying than any meal eaten at a famous restaurant or any other type of meal. The meals are also "healing injections". After eating a meal, a person feels alive, as if the meal itself is alive and emitting and transferring life. Every meal is a dose of "delicious medicine".

3. Comments about the book's non-restrictive approach to weight control. Here is a recapitulation of the compiled comments: Almost every diet book on the market is a "forbidding book". So many foods are forbidden, and so many frightening reasons given, that fear often accompanies one's efforts to

become healthy. Especially when one is dieting, fear becomes another word for diet. Dieting is forced, so a feeling of being tortured is forever present. One diet may force so much exercise, another so much water, then another near starvation. The feelings of being tortured are so overwhelming that one is impatient to get off that diet plan in order to lead a normal life again. But the minute one comes off that diet plan, one enjoys food even more and devours even more food than before. Because the desire for food is magnified when the body is starved, one quickly gains back all the weight that has been lost and more. The situation after dieting is even worse than before, and it steadily deteriorates until one is eager to get back on a diet plan again, however tortured one may feel. But then once on a diet plan, the cravings for food build again—with disastrous consequences. There is no end to the mental and physical suffering. So whenever one hears of a diet plan, one is gripped by fear. This book stops the suffering by allowing one to eat and lose weight at the same time. One gets the most satisfaction, without gaining one ounce in weight. When the diet becomes balanced, so does the person. And once the entire person becomes balanced, the sense of moderation naturally becomes a built-in power that prevents any overeating.

4. Statements against eating meat. Some vegetarians have been complaining that the book does not advocate vegetarianism. My argument is that vegetarianism is a practice that has its own geographical and resource conditional backgrounds. The central theme of Taoism is balance, so this book is about getting balanced nutrition, in a balanced and undiscriminating manner—that is, not at the expense of any one group of organisms.

In my opinion, plants do not deserve to be killed for food any more than animals do. According to the latest scientific research, plants react to the stimulus of touch, listen to music, sense stress at the death of other organisms, bleed, make the oxygen we breathe, and more. They provide adequate amounts of food and protection for their offspring until they have grown adequately enough to obtain food for themselves. They also get sick when they are infected by microscopic organisms, some of which are capable of infecting both plant and man. During a transplantation, plants suffer from root shock and undergo physiological changes that may lead to death. There is no doubt that plants, too, are living organisms. Being so, is killing plants more humane than killing animals? Or are the plants' silent screams less meaningful than the vocal screams of animals?

If we contemplated on what plants must endure when they are yanked out of the earth for food, we would have only air left to eat. But even that is filled with living organisms. Unknowingly and constantly, we breathe in millions of microorganisms which are later eliminated by our immune systems. We also kill millions of microorganisms harbored in the vegetables or meats we cook and eat, everyday. These microorganisms are essentially microscopic animals— some of them look like elephants under the microscope. Some have incredible and intricate modes and structures of movement—some have *muscles*. Some play very important roles in helping us digest, create, and absorb nutrients. Some are capable of synthesizing hormones (insulin for example) for human use. They have amazing and intricate structures for ingesting food, digesting food, and excreting food. Some even have reproductive actions reminiscent of those of human beings. For these and many other reasons, there can not be a pure vegetarian in the entire universe.

If my life is meaningless, then all the lives that have been lost to support it have been wasted; then I am a great sinner. If my life is meaningful, then I need other lives (food) to support it in order to accomplish my mission. According to Taoist theory, one meaning of life is to learn how to use all God-given resources well, in a responsible and balanced way, for the elevation of every organism. This lesson extends to all organisms, including man. (To a Taoist, every spark of life has its meaning, its purpose.) Taoists believe in the continuity of life. Just because the form of life changes does not mean that life itself discontinues—it continues on in another form. Once an organism serves it life purpose well, it has accumulated merits that allow it to continue on, to evolve to a more complex form. Evolution itself has a purpose, the study of which represents a separate and complex knowledge of its own and is not explained here. For further information, please read the book entitled *The Great Tao*.

Since this book is about balance, it neither recommends nor condemns vegetarianism. I myself like vegetables very much, but I do not think it is fair to force my opinion upon others. There are those who must expend a great deal of energy in daily life and therefore need meat to support them. So the book has pure meat and pure vegetable dishes. (There are many vegetable dishes to choose from.) In the selection of a dish, every individual must be true to his or her needs. For example, a person who does heavy physical work and eats vegetables only will be incapable. On the other hand, it would be foolish if a cardiac or diabetic patient ate great amounts of meat. But there is one constant rule: according to the universal health principle, we must combine meat with vegetables whenever we eat meat.

5. Questions about calorie counting. It is not mentioned in the book, because I think enough books on the subject of calorie counting have been written and another book on it is unnecessary. Even with so many books on calorie counting on the market, many people still come to me with weight problems. Therefore, calorie counting is not the answer to weight control, as it is not effective on a long-term basis. In my opinion, calorie counting causes the body to crave more foods with more calories, or worse, encourages the body to convert calories into fat. Constant calorie counting lowers the caloric intake, but it trains the body to become more efficient at utilizing whatever calories are available. Because calories are no longer abundant, the body utilizes or stores every calorie instead of passing it up. After a while, calorie counting loses its effectiveness and the body gains weight. The only way to fight this regression is to

cut out more calories, but in time even lower calorie counts can not produce satisfactory results. The calorie count must be lowered and lowered until finally nothing is eaten. From recent studies, it is now known that a constant state of deprivation causes the body to sacrifice its current energy needs to save energy for future use, in an effort to prolong life. The body saves energy by converting it into fat deposits. The result: a listless and overweight body. Furthermore, once calorie counting is begun, stopping it is difficult. The minute one stops calorie counting while the body functions at increased efficiency, the body will rapidly put on even more weight. Calorie counting also jeopardizes food balance; instead of making dietary balance the first priority, the calorie counter immerses him or herself in calorie totaling before food is eaten, and concern for balance is set aside or completely forgotten. Finally unfamiliarity with the caloric value of different foods may restrict the calorie counter to a limited selection of foods and deter him or her from eating balanced meals.

6. Questions about abstinence from sugar and salt. The book does not recommend abstinence from sugar or salt, even though nearly every nutritional/health/diet book warns against sugar and salt and every expert advises against eating sugar and salt. The reason again is balance. Sugar and salt are essential ingredients of balanced meals and, therefore, play important roles in health and weight control. Sugar and salt were not intended by God to be bad for humans. If sugar and salt were bad, the human race would have ended long ago. Proper use of sugar and salt—balanced use—will not result in problems; overuse and nonuse will. Overuse causes sugar and salt to be isolated as the causes of health problems. Nonuse results in not only nonfunctional internal organs, but also unenjoyable meals. And if one could not enjoy one's meals, one of the greatest joys of living would be gone. Furthermore, the Food and Drug Administration recently announced that, after thorough research, there was no evidence whatsoever linking sugar intake to obesity, di-

abetes, high blood pressure, hypersensitivity, or heart disease. To find out how to use sugar and salt properly, please read text. If modern methods of refining sugar offend the reader, please do not hesitate to use raw sugar or honey instead.

7. Questions about artificial vitamin and mineral supplements. Taking artificial vitamin and mineral supplements is not recommended in the book because vitamins and minerals are very young concepts. There is no one in the world who has a perfect knowledge of these supplements. Nevertheless, we need not worry about nutritional shortages, as long as we eat balanced foods—foods that nature made. Besides, according to the Five Tastes Theory and Energy Theory, food is not only composed of vitamins A, B, C, D, etc. It is also made up of living energy, healing powers, and so on. (More about vitamins and minerals later.)

8. Questions about basing one's diet solely on foods native to one's habitat. This is not recommended in the book for this reason: balance. No habitat can be so perfect as to yield all manner of spices, fruits, vegetables, poultry, etc. naturally. The selection would most certainly be limited and unbalanced. Therefore, restricting oneself to native foods is like purposely denying oneself balanced meals. Limiting one's diet is a rather difficult thing to do, especially in this age of global communication. The entire globe is one unit—the entire world shares the same sun, water, and soil. There are no natural boundaries, only political boundaries.

9. Questions about the seasonal concept of eating. This concept of eating is not practicable. For details please read text.

10. Questions about the itemization of the healing effectiveness of every food. This is not done because there are four qualities of regular foods that one can depend upon: good taste, good appearance, good aroma, and good nutrition—and healing properties are not among them. Since regular foods are used only for maintaining basic life, the healing powers of regular

foods are so minimal that one can not depend upon them for curative affects. The nutrient and effective property levels of regular foods are not high enough to correct diseases and rejuvenate and repair cells. Only herbs, called Forgotten Foods, contain sufficient nutrient and medicinal levels—and are powerful enough—to heal the body. A thorough explanation and itemization of herbal healing effectiveness is given in *The Great Tao*.

In appreciation for the attentiveness of the readers and the success of many thousands in achieving healthful balance, I wish to present this new hardcover edition. Revised and enriched, this edition is also offered in gratitude for the readers' generosity and patience regarding the first, paperback edition. Specifically: Their overlooking the brevity of the book. (As the first edition was intended only to be a handbook, some related subjects were overlooked.) Their overlooking the mistakes and typographical errors and determining for themselves the true meanings. Their overlooking the rapid wear and tear of the book from daily use. And their requests for slight design changes that allow the book to match their collection.

I hope this book will help every reader live longer, healthier, happier, and wiser.

Dr. Stephen T. Chang

PART I

1

Taoism

The Tao of Balanced Diet is about one part of the living philosophy of Taoism. It is about one of the Eight Pillars, or eight branches, of Taoist thought and practice. These Eight Pillars are symbolized as eight trigrams in the *Pa-Kua* symbol of Taoism.

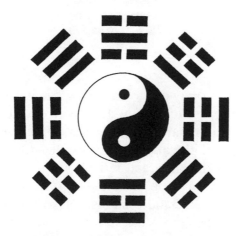

Figure 1. Pa-Kua (Symbol of Taoism). The eight trigrams (pointing in 8 different directions from the Yin-Yang symbol) represent the Eight Pillars of Taoism.

Many true Taoist teachings have been kept secret for many centuries, so before we begin examining the Theory of Balanced Diet in detail, the Eight Pillars will be listed and then briefly summarized.

1. The Tao of Philosophy
2. The Tao of Revitalization (Internal Exercises)
3. The Tao of Balanced Diet
4. The Tao of Forgotten Food Diet
5. The Tao of Healing Art
6. The Tao of Sex Wisdom
7. The Tao of Mastery
8. The Tao of Success

THE TAO OF PHILOSOPHY

The Tao of Philosophy discloses the logic underlying the way life unfolds and the purpose of destiny. It is a collection of guidelines that is used by the individual as well as the collectivity for attaining success and spiritual elevation. Based on the spiritual discovery of hidden but ever-permeating and reliable laws of this universe, the Tao of Philosophy provides detailed information on the proper methods of government and fosterage of social development and individual well-being.

THE TAO OF REVITALIZATION

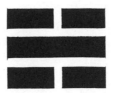

The Tao of Revitalization, also called Internal Exercises, are divided into three categories.

The first category of Internal Exercises includes those designed to direct the innate healing power to specific internal organs and glands to energize the entire body, balance the energy level, and promote a more effective functioning of the internal organs, in order to heal, adjust, correct, and above all prevent disease. These exercises are the Five Animal Exercises, Eight Directional Exercises, Twelve Zodiac Exercises, and Twelve Nerve Exercises. Also included are the basic exercises known as the Deer Exercise, the Crane Exercise, and the Turtle Exercise, used for correcting sex-related problems, digestive and weight problems, and nerve-related problems.

The second category includes Meridian Meditation, also known as Trip-Around-the-World Meditation, or simply Taoist Contemplation. A tremendous healing art, Meridian Meditation is used to adjust, balance, and elevate the energy level in the body. By meditating on the pathways of energy in the body, anatomically known as the meridians, a person is able to feel the energy flow along these pathways and balance the energies within the body. The mind, body, and spirit are completely integrated, and the individual is completely enlivened. (Acupuncture and acupressure techniques, which originated from Meridian Meditation, are used to help others, whereas Meridian Meditation is used to heal oneself.)

The third category of Internal Exercises concerns energy breathing techniques. Through these techniques, energy can be absorbed through the acupuncture points which lie atop the meridians which traverse the body. Energy breathing is a vital step in self-healing and in forming an indivisible link with the energy permeating the universe.

In sum, the main purpose of the Internal Exercises is to promote longevity.

THE TAO OF BALANCED DIET

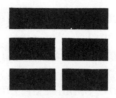

This is the subject of this book, the purpose of which is to explain clearly the complete theory and practice of the Tao of Balanced Diet.

THE TAO OF FORGOTTEN FOOD DIET

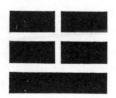

We rely on our regular diet for enjoyment and satisfaction: we take pleasure in the appearance, aroma, and taste of our daily meals. But regular foods do not provide enough nutrients to maintain a continuous state of health. They must be supplemented with stronger foods, or herbal foods, which constitute the second level of diet, or Tao of Forgotten Food Diet.

Over the ages, Taoists thoroughly studied the healing composition of herbs and became highly proficient at the use of herbs. For example, several thousand years ago, surgeons were able to anesthetize their patients for six hours without side-effects just by using an herb tea. (Surgery was very popular at that time. The surgeons often removed the organs of the patient, washed them in herbal solutions, and reorganized them inside the body. This practice eventually died out as these doctors came to realize that it was an inefficient and incomplete treatment for diseases and that the final answer lay in disease prevention. They realized that any illness, including tumors, was the result of a particular lifestyle; constant surgery could not prevent the recurrence of tumors, whereas a change in lifestyle could.)

Herbs have many properties that modern science has yet to discover. The Academy of Sciences currently estimates that there are approximately one million plant varieties in the world. As yet, only an insignificant portion has been examined by modern means of analysis.

The food we buy in the supermarket is the weakest food available. The selection there is very limited if one considers the varieties of food actually available in the world. God created leaves, branches, trunks, and roots for our consumption, but they were completely overlooked by most people. Called "Forgotten Foods" by Taoists, herbs were forgotten because they were eliminated from our ancestors' diets through a process of selection which, over the course of thousands of years, rejected foods that were unappealing to the eyes, nose, or mouth. When man learned to cultivate his own food, he naturally chose to cultivate only those foods that appealed to his senses. As the saying goes, we are what we eat. If we eat stronger foods, we become stronger ourselves. If we eat better foods, our health improves. But, if we eat weak foods, we become more vulnerable to diseases. When we compare a magnolia tree to a bunch of celery, we will see that the tree is much stronger than the little clump of celery. Investigating further, we will find that the tree is of greater medicinal value than the celery. In fact, the various properties of the magnolia tree build up the stomach tissues and strengthen the female sexual organs. Ginseng is another example of a strong food. It grows in cold and harsh mountainous regions, yet it can survive for more than a thousand years. Imagine what such great vitality could do for your body! (Please use discretion when ingesting ginseng. It must be balanced with other herbs, since it produces strong side-effects as well as benefits.) In sharp contrast, a carrot grows only in temperate climates and its lifespan is about three months. If you do not unearth it within three months, it will decay and disappear. Herbs give everlasting strength, whereas regular foods give only temporary strength.

The foods we commonly eat and love are also eaten and loved by the germs in our bodies. They utilize this food (organic or junk) to maintain their lives just as we do. Fortunately, herbs do not nourish germs and human beings equally. Human beings, exercising their will power, are able to ingest sometimes distasteful herbs. Germs, not being blessed with will power, are simply repelled by herbs. When human blood is permeated with herbal nutrients, the germs in the body will starve , and the human body will be naturally cleansed and purified. The cleansing and purifying qualities that allow herbs to last for years without rotting are the greatest benefits to be gained from herbal diets.

THE TAO OF HEALING ART

Like the Tao of Revitalization, the Tao of Healing Art adjusts, balances and elevates vital energy. Unlike the Tao of Revitalization, which is primarily a means for self- healing, the Tao of Healing Art is utilized for healing others.

The Tao of Healing Art, also called Tui-Na, is basically a form of massage that follows the body's energy pathways, anatomically known as meridians, to regulate the body's vital functions. By using the sixteen different handling or manipulating techniques of Tui-Na, one can also reposition disarranged internal organs. In conjunction with these techniques, which were designed to adapt to various parts of the body, appropriate mediums can also be used. These can belong to any of the five fundamental "elements" of the universe: earth, metal, water, wood, or fire. Acupuncture needles (used to channel energy into the body) and moxibustion are two of the best known metal and fire mediums in the West. (Acupuncture and moxibustion are derivations of Tui-Na principles and methods.) For more information, please refer to *The Great Tao*, Chapter 5.

THE TAO OF SEX WISDOM

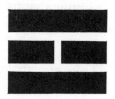

Taoism was the first philosophy to take human sexuality fully into account, to present it in such a way that people could use their sexual energy to transform themselves. Taoist Sexology directs people so they can enjoy sexual play without depleting themselves, explains how to strengthen the sexual organs and use sexual energy to cure specific ailments, strengthens the bond of love, elucidates various positions of therapeutic intercourse, even provides natural methods of family planning and eugenics.

THE TAO OF MASTERY

The Tao of Mastery provides us with tools to help us gain insight into ourselves and others, bend surrounding forces to our nature and purpose, and become masters of ourselves.

In order to facilitate personal and working relationships and reduce stress, the ancient Taoists developed a collection of different methods:

1. PERSONOLOGY reveals the current abilities, attitudes, personal traits, and health conditions of an individual. Instinctive anticipation of forthcoming events is reflected in some of the 108 locations of the face, constituting a recognizable warning system.

2. FINGERPRINT SYSTEM reveals the inherited part of personality and health tendencies. Also, fingerprints are changing delineations of our naturally developing personal and professional potentials and are warning signals of our inherited weaknesses, which we must be aware of in order to conquer them.

3. TAOIST NUMEROLOGY gives precise insights into our life patterns and circumstances.

4. NORTH STAR ASTROLOGICAL SYSTEM—more comprehensive and scientific than Western astrology—reveals our destinies and financial prospects; describes the physical, mental, and spiritual attributes of our spouse and children; and unveils all other facets of our lives.

5. DIRECTIONOLOGY is the study of the surrounding physical laws of nature, especially those of electromagnetism. A complete knowledge of such forces allows us to orient ourselves and our belongings in ways compatible with the electromagnetic influences, in order to live in harmony with the laws of nature and facilitate obtainment of goals. On the collective level, it can be used to reduce in-fighting and promote the "chemistry" or cooperation between workers. It is used in modern Japan to organize working groups as well as coordinate the various departments of a company. In the West, the awareness of these influences is reflected in conversations about the "ambience" or the "morale" at working places.

6. SYMBOLOGY deals with forms and symbols related to the laws underlying natural events. It can be used to condition, for instance, weather changes, business trends, self-defeating habits, etc.

THE TAO OF SUCCESS

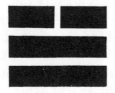

The Tao of Success discloses the precise mechanics of life's greatest events and the forces that shape all events. The ancient Taoists discovered analytical methods to study these forces, identified recognizable patterns of change, and systematized strategies of success to deal with these patterns. The Tao of Success helps you adjust your everyday actions in accordance with the universal law, to make every aspect of life more pleasant.

A clear and powerful instrument of Taoist wisdom, the Tao of Success is divided into three parts:

1. The study of symbols and signs that represent the endless changes that occur throughout the universe. These phenomena are governed by exact laws defined by physics, chemistry, biology, geometry, algebra, and other branches of mathematics.

2. The Tao of Change, or the study of social philosophy and transactional psychology, as represented by sixty-four hexagrams. Each hexagram is composed of six lines, each of which represents a developing stage in individual or group transactions. Recognition of a certain pattern allows one to develop successful, detailed, and accurate strategies against the causes of adversity. The Tao of Change is invaluable to those who wish to develop wealth, power, harmonious familial relations, social position, and foresight fully.

3. The actual practice of forecasting events, known as the Space and Time I-Ching System. This system is based on the principle of cyclicalness—that is, everything that has happened is going to happen again, and everything that is going to happen has happened already in some form. Like Albert Einstein, the ancient Taoists understood that time was illusory. Like him, they studied situations in the space-time system. Thus, they arrived at a means for interpreting events occurring within our time concept. This is the key to "forecasting", or seeing into the future.

The Eight Pillars of Taoism cover every aspect of our daily existence. They were designed to completely satisfy our basic physical needs in a manner that allows us to realize our full potential as human beings. Then may we leap beyond the degenerating aspect of time, to live with the Tao, or God.

2

Obesity

THE RESULTS OF OBESITY

There is no need for anyone to be overweight. Nor is there a need to be underweight. In fact, from the point of view of Taoism—the 6,000 year old Chinese philosophy and science of life—there is basically no difference between being overweight or underweight. Both reflect a lack of balance in the human being. In Taoism, every being in the universe is considered to have its own center, and all parts of the being should be in balance with this center. In a human being weight is one aspect of this balance. Each person has a proper weight depending on his or her height, bone structure, shape and other factors. If you are over or under your proper weight, you are out of balance. And because a human being is more than just a physical body, weight imbalance indicates that your spiritual and mental bodies are imbalanced also.

Because of the diet and lifestyle in the Western world, obesity is the major weight imbalance in our society. It is present in all degrees, from extreme obesity to "slightly overweight". You might think that a few extra pounds make no difference. But those few pounds appear different when we realize that for every inch of excess fatty tissue on our bodies, we need an additional *four miles* of blood vessels to support that tissue. And that requires your heart to work harder, pumping blood through that four miles of blood vessels. Two inches of excess tissue require eight miles of blood vessels, three inches need twelve miles. Twelve more miles through which your heart has to pump blood. That is a great deal of extra work for your heart. And that extra strain is going to weaken your heart, and eventually cause it to break down.

It is no different than with an automobile. If you load your car too heavily and use it for a long time under the additional strain, the engine will break down. As the heart—your engine—is over-worked, it becomes enlarged. The muscles soften and loosen. It no longer has the strength it formerly had. As it deteriorates, it becomes more susceptible to germs, viruses, bacteria, and other organisms which can attack weak muscles of the heart and cause inflammation. When a heart attack occurs, even if not fatal, it results in the "death" of one area of the heart tissue—it is no longer capable of functioning. A second heart attack results in the "death" of another area of the heart. This increases the strain on the still-functioning parts of the heart, which must work harder to maintain the activity of the circulatory system. Fortunately, from a thousand year study we know there are herbs which can provide the right type of nutrition to regenerate new heart cells. But there is no reason for you to need them in the first place. Because there is no reason to be overweight.

Another result of obesity—and its resulting hardening of the arteries and weakened heart—is high blood pressure. Standard medical procedure is for a doctor to prescribe pills to reduce your blood pressure. These pills *do* reduce your blood pressure. They do this by opening your arteries and allowing your blood to flow more freely. But your heart will continue to work as hard as ever—*undetected* by the blood pressure monitor—because the basic cause, water retention, is unresolved. The pills satisfy the machine, not the body. In addition, blood pressure pills weaken the kidneys. This results in water retention which leads to blocked circulation, which again results in a weakened heart and blood vessels, which cause more high blood pressure. To assist the kidneys, your doctor will prescribe diuretics. Unfortunately, diuretics have the opposite effect which doctors hope for; they further weaken the kidneys, lead to increased water retention and shortage of potassium, which result in high blood pressure. It becomes a vicious circle, with one "cure" causing another problem, eventually worsening the illness the medicine was supposed to cure. And all of this is taking place in your body, at the expense of your health.

Gallstones are another result of obesity. Composed of hard, dried fat—almost like rubber—they are very hard to dissolve. You can also find yourself more susceptible to hypoglycemia or diabetes, both results of a weak pancreas, an organ weakened by obesity.

In China, most diseases resulting from obesity are called "diseases of the rich". So obesity and the diseases and health problems associated with it are results of material success. But these problems are not necessary. It is possible to live in a society such as ours, enjoy its benefits, and still avoid the diseases which its excesses lead to. To do this we must first know exactly what causes excessive weight. Then we must know how to reduce it. This book will tell you all you need to know about both areas in order to have a healthy, well-balanced body, and the long, vigorous life you deserve.

THE EIGHT CAUSES OF WEIGHT PROBLEMS

1. Self-Poisoning

If the food you eat does not have the proper pH balance—that is, acid-alkaline balance—it can putrefy in your stomach before your body gets a chance to digest it and absorb its nutrients. In other words, before you eat it, the harmful organisms in your stomach get it first. *They* digest it, and leave you their wastes. The wastes include gas—which you will notice through bad breath, belching, flatulence, or stomach pains—and solids, which are of no nutritional value to your body. They do not provide the nutrients your cells need, your cells become weaker as a result, and these waste products—literally poisons—cannot be eliminated, resulting in the cells of your entire body being poisoned. The only way to prevent this type of self-poisoning is through a properly balanced diet, because the proper pH balance works as a natural preservative to prevent putrefaction, corruption, and decay of foods in your stomach. (See p.95-97 for detailed information on pH balancing.)

2. Water Retention

The kidneys are the filters that separate waste water from the blood. So the amount of water filtered out depends on how well your kidneys are functioning. Normal kidneys can filter approximately six cups of water in twenty-four hours. (It is possible for them to filter a larger volume but this requires them to work harder, and the increased strain eventually weakens them.)

So if your kidneys are normal, you can drink six cups of water a day and you will break even. But, if you drink *more* than what your kidneys can handle—and remember: for most people the limit is six cups a day!—this water will remain in your body. It will travel back into the blood stream to be eliminated through the skin by perspiration. However, if you have few opportunities to perspire (cold weather, no exercise, etc.), the water will be retained in your skin. As more and more waste water comes to the area of your skin where water is already being retained, the tissue in that area bloats up to receive the incoming water. This "stagnant" water remains, retaining even more wastes and associated toxins. This accumulated waste water—considered as *urine*—may stay in this area for a day, a month, even a year or more. After a period of time, this water becomes mucus. This mucus is still waste water, only it is in a more solid form. You may think you have added fat. But it is simply mucus which is stuck between the tissues. When this gelatinous substance hardens sufficiently, we call it *cellulite*. Animal fats such as butter and lard are particular components of cellulite formation. *And you will not get rid of cellulite by exercise or perspiration alone*—only "fresh" water is eliminated by perspiration. The only way is by:

1. Drinking less—limiting your daily liquid intake to less than 6 cups—this is very important.

2. Manipulating the cellulite deposits, preferably in a sauna or hot bath.

The secret of cellulite manipulation is to "heat up and break up" the deposits. The more you deeply massage these deposits, the more they can break up and be eliminated. The heat also causes the pores to open to allow increased perspiration.

When we talk about a limit of six cups of liquid in twenty-four hours, we mean *all* liquids, including soup, beverages, fruit and vegetables. You cannot eat two big bowls of soup and say that you did not drink any water. You can still retain water from that soup, so it must be acknowledged.

For example, one patient of mine was overweight. He ate only one actual meal a day. The rest of the time he drank fruit juices. He had no idea how many gallons of liquids he actually poured into his body. Because he lived on almost nothing but fruit juice, he received almost no nutrients. Because of this lack of nutrition, he was very weak, constantly fainted, had palpitations of the heart, was short of breath, and had gout! (Chinese medicine indicates that gout is a symptom of kidney problems.) He also had high blood pressure. He had these problems for years, but he never made the connection between his symptoms and his "healthful" fruit juice diet.

Often people will go to a restaurant, order a large salad and a glass of water, and congratulate themselves on their self-discipline. They think they are losing weight. But all they are doing is cheating themselves. Chances are that their kidneys are not functioning 100%, so the more water they drink, the more will be retained in their bodies. So the more liquids they take in—even in that salad—the more weight they gain.

How well are your kidneys functioning? You can determine that by following these guidelines:

1. If your body has cellulite, there is no doubt that your kidneys are not functioning 100%, because you are retaining water. To check for cellulite, check the areas around the buttocks, thighs, belly, and upper arms for flabby or jelly-like tissues under the skin.

2. If you experience rapid weight changes—that is, gaining or losing as much as five pounds in a period of a day or two—those weight changes are definitely retained water, not fat. No fatty tissues can come and go that quickly.

3. If, when you press down with your finger on your arm or leg for a moment, then withdraw it, you see a white impression on your skin which remains briefly, you have water retention. If no water is being retained, there is either no white mark, or it disappears immediately. The longer it stays, the greater the water retention problem.

4. If your physician diagnoses your weight problem as water retention, unfortunately the standard medical cure for water retention is diuretic pills. I call these "beat your tired horse" pills. Why? Because your horse (your kidneys) is already "tired"—that is why you are retaining water. Taking these pills makes your "horse" run even harder. Overnight you may lose 10 pounds. The problem is that when you take these pills, you have to drink more water to wash them down. In fact, your doctor will tell you to drink great quantities of water in order to lubricate and "flush out" your kidneys. So you end up taking in (and eventually retaining) as much or more water than you eliminate. And during the process, you work your kidneys even harder, making them weaker and less capable of functioning properly. Ultimately, overworking your kidneys this way will cause kidney disease or even total failure. We live in a "drinking country". Most people have a high daily intake of liquids. So it is not surprising that we also have a high incidence of

kidney disease. But now that you know better, you can escape the norm—and stay healthy by decreasing the amount of liquids you drink.

3. Accumulation of Fat

Fats are related to the pancreas and liver functions, and also to the gallbladder function. The liver is the main organ of the body for filtering out solid wastes. Since the poisons and toxins in our bodies are in solid form, we need lubrication to carry them out. Fats provide this lubrication. so it is necessary for us to eat fat.

The problem occurs once the fat is absorbed into the blood stream and carried to the liver. If the amount of fat is excessive, or the structure of the fat is such that it cannot be easily broken down by the body, it will clog the liver tissues, blocking part of the liver's proper functions. Since the liver's function has been partially blocked, more of the wastes cannot be filtered out. This eventually leads to poisoning of the brain and nerve cells by toxins in the blood stream, leading to disorders we call nervous and mental problems—just some of the many detrimental effects of a poorly functioning liver.

Fats can also accumulate in certain parts of the body which are seldom exercised, such as the stomach and hips. When this happens a person begins to accumulate more and more fat. As a result it becomes harder to breathe, and breathing may become quite short and shallow. Fat accumulation also affects the heart, causing palpitations (rapid and irregular heartbeat), fibrillation (uneven contraction of the heart), or skipping pulse. Skipping pulse occurs when the heart muscles are loaded down with fat, or when the blood is too thick to flow smoothly. All of these problems are caused by accumulated fats.

Since we do need fats in our diet, what kind should we eat? Animal fat is the most difficult for our livers to deal with. This is particularly true of beef fat, including butter, because it cannot be metabolized by our bodies. Few people realize that margarine is even worse. In the process of making margarine it is heated to a very high temperature, making its chemical structure very strong and very difficult for the body temperature to break down.

The best type of fat to use is vegetable oil. And the best type of vegetable oil is sesame oil, or any other oil that you can rinse off your fingers without using a detergent.

In case you have no choice and must consume more fat (animal *and* vegetable) than necessary, you can alleviate problems by drinking strong tea. It must be a type of tea that contains a natural detergent to "wash out" the excess fat, but if it is unavailable, a cup of Lipton tea is better than nothing. Hundreds of years ago, Taoists developed a tea for this purpose, using chrysanthemum flowers (for its detergent qualities) and honeysuckle flowers (for its antibiotic qualities), and have been drinking it ever since with their meals.

4. Nerves

Allergies result when the nerve endings cannot tolerate a particular food, or substance in a food. If you are allergic to some type of food, you cannot digest it. If you cannot digest it, it becomes "poisonous" to you. This toxic (to you) food then adds to your weight problem. (See Weight Cause #1—Self-Poisoning.) Also, foods that you crave are poisonous to you, so you should be especially cautious.

Another aspect of nerves as a cause of obesity are eating habits resulting from nervousness. One type is the person who has become lazy. He or she just sits and thinks about things that need to be done. Of course, they never do it. They then become guilty about not doing what is needed to be done and become even more nervous. So they get no exercise, and eat continually to try to forget their guilt about their inactivity. It is a vicious circle. The worse they feel, the more they eat, the harder it is to do anything, and the worse they feel. The only solution is to do something. Anything. Some activity which will keep them busy. But of course they have to first overcome all mental hurdles, the excuses created about why anything cannot be done. It is not an easy position to be in. Or get out of.

5. Sexual Dissatisfaction

With women, sexual satisfaction depends on the man. Despite all the theories (and validity) of women's liberation, a woman's real sexual satisfaction physiologically relies on the man. According to Taoist theory, there are nine stages through which a woman must pass to reach a true climax. If a man cannot bring a woman through these stages, she will not be satisfied. (She will not be able to bring herself through these stages either.) And the more unsatisfied she is, the more nervous she becomes. The more nervous, the more she eats.

The following stages describe the complete cycle which will allow for total satisfaction.

Stage	*Energized Organ(s)*	*Observable Response*
One	Lungs	The woman sighs, breathes heavily, and salivates.
Two	Heart	The woman, while kissing the man, extends her tongue out to him. According to Su Wen, or Classic of the Internal by the Yellow Emperor, the tongue corresponds to the heart.
Three	Spleen, Pancreas and Stomach	As her muscles become activated, the woman grasps and holds the man tightly.
Four	Kidneys and Bladder	Women experience a series of vaginal spasms at this time and secretions begin to flow.
Five	Bones	The woman's joints loosen and she begins to bite the man.
Six	Liver and Nerves	The woman undulates and gyrates like a snake, trying to wrap her arms and legs around the man.

Seven	Blood	The woman's blood is "boiling", and she is frantically trying to touch the man everywhere.
Eight	Muscles	Her muscles totally relax. She bites even more and grabs the man's nipples.
Nine	The entire body is energized.	She collapses in a "little death". She completely surrenders to the man and is completely opened up.

For a woman to be completely satisfied, a man must carry her through all nine of these stages. Most men carry women only through the fourth stage, then roll over and go to sleep. Many men, even women, mistake the vaginal spasm at Level Four for a complete orgasm. But as you can see, that is not even half of a complete orgasm. Unfortunately, most sex manuals support the former view, because the observable responses at the fourth level are considered as the total orgasm. So the woman is trapped halfway. She cannot "go to heaven" or "go down to earth". Even masturbation cannot give her the full psychological experience of the last four stages. So she sleeps fitfully all night. At daybreak her partner wakes her up and tells her to make breakfast. She tells him to do it himself, because she has a headache. They both start the day angry and feel irritable all day long. Finally they break up. Meanwhile she is filled with nervous tension and overeats. And she ends up with a weight problem as well.

6. Overeating and Overdrinking

These neurotic manifestations can result from psychological programming in childhood. Most adults, when they were children, were encouraged—or even told—to eat "more" or drink "more" by their parents, because their parents loved them and wanted them to grow "big and healthy". The beliefs and opinions of the parents gradually sunk into the child's subconscious. As the child grew up, he felt guilty when he did not eat or consume enough. So he developed an unconscious habit to eat, eat, eat, or drink, drink, drink. The result—obesity.

7. Five Morphological Types

According to Taoist theory, there are five basic morphological types—Metal, Earth, Wood, Water and Fire—of human beings. The five morphological types and their characteristics are as follows:

Morphological Type   *Characteristics*

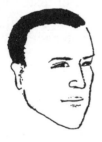

Charismatic, intelligent, comely, sharp-featured, confident, self-indulgent, selfish, superficial.

a. Metal

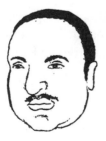

Practical, frugal, thick-skinned, business-oriented, thick and tight musculature.

b. Earth

Figures 2a—2e. The Five Morphological Types.

41

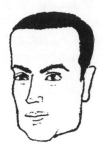

Stubborn, thin and bony,
deep-thinking, fastidious,
unhurried, unchanging.

c. Wood

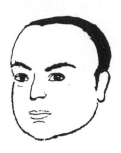

Flexible, unstabilized,
clever, critical, super-
ficially easy-going, soft
and water retentive tissues.

d. Water

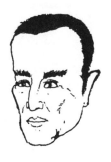

Quick-tempered, nervous,
forward, extremely bright,
creative, talented.

e. Fire

Figures 2a—2e continued.

The two morphological types most likely to appear overweight are Earth and Water. This is the normal condition for these individuals. If their bodies are chiseled into another form with diets, exercise, etc., they will not feel happy or content with themselves, as they are thrown off balance mentally and physically. Recent research confirms that for some overweight individuals, the overweight condition is normal, while any condition below that point of normality can cause mental and physical problems. In contrast, there are some people for whom extreme thinness is normal. Their morphological type is Wood. Regardless of one's weight, it is more important to maintain a state of normality, or balance, because it is the basis for health, happiness, contentment, and longevity. And the theories of dietary balance put forth in this book are designed to do so.

8. Health Problems

Heart disease, thyroid dysfunction, pancreas disorder, adrenal and thymus gland disorders—all can lead to obesity. These problems and diseases must be treated first before any attempt can be made to reduce weight.

Also, cortisone, aspirin, and other drugs used to relieve the pain of rheumatism, bronchitis, and asthma can lead to obesity. In fact obesity is a common side effect of the use of these drugs. In the first place drugs such as aspirin are acidic in themselves. Secondly, they cause the stomach to secrete more acid. Because the sensation of hunger occurs when the stomach acids have dissolved all the food in the stomach, the more acid, the more hunger. The more hunger, the more a person eats in an attempt to satisfy this hunger. And gradually the eating itself becomes a habit.

Note: Cortisone and other drugs used to treat these disorders can ruin the kidneys and other organs by causing them to lose their ability to function properly. If the function of the kidneys decreases, water will be retained and the process leading to an overweight condition begins again.

PART II

PART II

3

The Taoist Seven Ways of Weight Loss

We have seen all the ways in which we can put on excess weight. Now let us look at how we can take off that weight—in a safe, healthy, sensible way—based on practices that have been proven effective for over 6,000 years.

DISCIPLINE

To maintain good health and balanced weight, it is necessary to exercise discipline in eating habits.

YOU MUST EAT FOOD THREE TIMES A DAY ON A REGULAR SCHEDULE. IF YOU DO THIS, YOU WILL NEVER OVEREAT.

When you eat three times a day, you will always have something in your stomach, and you will not overeat out of excessive hunger at the next meal. So you must take a few days to develop this new habit of eating, but it will be well worth the effort. If breakfast is at 8:00 in the morning, then you must eat at 8:00 in the morning. If lunch is at noon, eat at noon. And if dinner is at 6:00 in the evening, eat at 6:00. NEVER MISS IT—for there is nothing more important than keeping to your schedule.

SUPPLEMENTAL HERBAL FORMULAS

Herbal combinations can be used to increase metabolism in the human body. Metabolism is controlled by the thyroid gland, which needs special nutrients to keep healthy and to function properly. Seaweed, for example, supplies a good amount of the nutrients the thyroid gland needs. Other herbs which are well known for their ability to improve metabolism, circulation, and detoxification are: Bupleurum, Pinellia, Scutellaria, Paeonia, Jujube, Rhubarb, Ginger, and Gardinia. Remember: All herbs *must* be used in a combination. When used alone they may have deleterious side effects.

In order to determine which herbal combinations are the best, it is recommended that you contact a knowledgeable physician or herbologist. The proper formula for each individual depends on the cause of the over- or underweight condition.

Shown below are a few examples of well-known herbal formulas.

Detoxifying Tea BP-404

Ingredients	Meridian Affected	Energy Characteristic	Taste
Bupleurum	Liver, Gallbladder	Cold	Bitter
Pinellia	Spleen-Pancreas, Stomach	Warm	Piquant
Poria	Heart, Lung, Spleen-Pancreas, Kidney	Neutral	Sweet
Cinnamon	Lung, Heart, Bladder	Hot	Sweet, Piquant
Scute	Heart, Lung, Gallbladder, Large and Small Intestines	Cold	Bitter
Jujube	Spleen-Pancreas, Stomach	Warm	Sweet
Ginger	Lung, Spleen-Pancreas Stomach	Warm	Piquant
Ginseng	Lung, Spleen-Pancreas	Warm	Sweet
Dragon Bone	Liver, Heart, Kidney	Neutral	Sweet
Oyster	Liver, Kidney	Cold	Salty
Rheum	Spleen-Pancreas, Stomach Large Intestine, Heart-Constrictor, Liver	Cold	Bitter

Benefits

This combination strengthens the liver. It is effective against fatigue, heart palpitation, insomnia, bed-wetting, hair loss, impotence, weak nerves (neurasthenia), prostatitis, and indigestion. It also helps stop smoking, drug addiction, and alcoholism. And it helps control weight.

Reducing Tea WD-307

Ingredients	Meridian Affected	Energy Characteristic	Taste
Bupleurum	Liver, Gallbladder	Cold	Bitter
Pinellia	Spleen-Pancreas, Stomach	Warm	Spicy
Scute	Heart, Lung, Gallbladder, Large and Small Intestines	Cold	Bitter
Paeonia	Liver, Spleen-Pancreas, Stomach	Cool	Sour, Bitter
Jujube	Spleen-Pancreas, Stomach	Warm	Sweet
Chih-Shih	Large Intestine, Lung	Cold	Bitter
Ginger	Lung, Spleen-Pancreas, Stomach	Warm	Spicy
Rhubarb	Spleen-Pancreas, Stomach, Large Intestine, Heart-Constrictor, Liver	Cold	Bitter

Benefits

This combination is used to adjust digestion, improve metabolism and eliminate congestion, reduce blood pressure, fight cholesterol and fatty materials, and improve elimination. It is well known as an obesity remedy and a preventive of obesity, and it can be used when the person suffers from constipation. This formula is not indicated in case of diarrhea.

Water Tea WD-302

Ingredients	Meridian Affected	Energy Characteristic	Taste
Alisma	Kidney, Bladder	Cold	Sweet
Polyporus	Kidney, Bladder	Neutral	Sweet
Poria	Heart, Lung, Spleen-Pancreas, Kidney	Neutral	Sweet
Atroctylodes	Spleen-Pancreas, Stomach	Warm	Sweet, Bitter
Cinnamon	Lung, Heart, Bladder	Warm	Sweet, Spicy

Benefits

This combination is used to strengthen the kidney and bladder and encourage metabolism. It is very effective for water retention and cellulite. It adjusts hormone levels and reduces blood pressure. It is also good for detoxification, headaches, menstrual problems, skin troubles, hair loss, and eye infections.

Regeneration Tea WD-301

Ingredients	Meridian Affected	Energy Characteristic	Taste
Rehmannia	Heart, Liver, Kidney	Cold	Sweet
Corus	Liver, Kidney	Warm	Sour
Dioscorea	Heart, Spleen-Pancreas, Kidney	Neutral	Sweet
Alisma	Kidney, Bladder	Cold	Sweet
Poria	Heart, Lung, Spleen-Pancreas, Kidney	Neutral	Sweet
Peony (tree)	Heart, Liver, Kidney	Cold	Bitter, Spicy
Cinnamon	Lung, Heart, Bladder	Hot	Sweet, Spicy
Aconite	Heart, Kidney, Spleen-Pancreas	Hot	Sweet, Spicy

Benefits

This interesting herbal combination, used in the East today for the treatment of diabetes, was developed 2,500 years ago for Emperor Han Wu-Ti, who had contracted the disease. Diabetes was officially recorded in Chinese medical history in the seventh century, approximately 1,000 years before its official discovery in the West.

This formula is good for adjusting blood sugar levels, regenerating the pancreas, kidney problems, kidney stones, bladder infections, nephritis (inflammation of the kidney), prostatitis, cataract, ringing in the ears, stopping hemorrhage, reducing blood pressure, and impotence.

The Japanese doctors have had magnificent results using this formula to treat the disease of senile cataract. For example, in 1957, Sigenari Ogura, M.D., started to treat patients for senile cataracts with this formula. He compiled a report on 41 cases. Among the 82 eyes treated, the visual power of 68 (83%) improved. Eight (10%) remained unchanged and 6 (7%) decreased. Ken Fujihira, M.D., reported the complete data of 285 senile cataract cases treated with this formula at his clinic between January 1 and December 31, 1975. His results showed that 172 (60.2%) improved. Thirty- four (12%) were unchanged, 29 (10.2%) were unstable (unstable meaning vision improving in one eye while worsening in another), 50 (17.6%) worsened (the total number improved and unchanged is 206, or 72.2%).

INTERNAL EXERCISES FOR VIGOR, HEALTH, AND THINNESS

The Internal Exercises were developed thousands of years ago in ancient China. They are designed to prevent disease, maintain good health, and increase longevity. Many of them are specifically recommended for weight reduction.

The Internal Exercises differ greatly from the *external exercises* done in the West. While external exercises such as football, boxing, aerobics, gymnastics, weight-lifting, Hatha Yoga, and martial arts may produce an attractive outer figure, they often do so by depleting the energy of the internal organs, thereby causing not only any number of illnesses, but also premature aging. The fatigue, stress, strain, pain, and contortions associated with the external exercises disrupt the delicate organic functions. Since responsibility for the body's regenerative processes and defenses against disease-causing agents lies in the internal organs, disrupting their functions will impair the body's ability to replace old or worn cells and fight off germs and viruses. The internal organs do what thick muscles can not do: protect the body against age and disease. Fortunately these organ functions are protected by the Internal Exercises, which adjust, energize, and heal the organs. And when internal organs are healthy, attractive figures naturally result.

What are going to be discussed in the following pages are disarmingly simple methods of losing weight and inches. The same methods or exercises also promotes clear thinking, proper digestion, sound sleep, and a healthy heart, to name a few benefits. Of course, all these things are related. The simple fact of being overweight has complex ramifications throughout a person's body. I will examine the most important of those ramifications and effects in this text, but before I do so I must give you some background information.

As a person gets older, exercising the stomach and abdominal area becomes increasingly difficult. It is not a very good idea to be doing sit ups after the age of forty, unless you are now, and have been, engaged in a regular exercise program for some time. The problem is that, unlike most of the other bodily extremities, the abdominal area cannot be directly controlled. (There are, however, thoroughly documented cases of advanced yogis who have perfect control over even these so-called "involuntary muscles".) Such men are the exceptions to the rule. For the rest of us, deposits of various kinds and fatty tissue accumulate there very easily.

But the conventional methods for losing weight and inches are quite often not only very difficult, but also very expensive!

So the simplest and most natural ways of losing weight and inches are the Deer Exercise, the Crane Exercise and its derivatives— the Solar Plexus Exercise and Stomach Rubbing Exercise—the Turtle Exercise, and Weight Reduction Exercise. With the practice of these exercises the peripheral and central causes of weight imbalance are corrected, almost without effort. In the Crane and related exercises, for instance, only gentle massaging of the abdomen and feelings are involved. The hand moves around gently, massaging the intestines, the blood vessels, and the digestive and eliminatory system. Fatty accumulations and deposits are disturbed from their resting places and eventually broken up. They are then passed into the eliminatory system and out of the body. By such apparently simple means, the superfluous areas of the stomach and abdomen are literally rubbed away!

What is really taking place while you are rubbing your stomach away is this: When the hand is gently passed over the body, energy invisible to the unaided eye passes from the hand into and through the skin. So when you move your hand around, you are actually "brushing" the cells and tissues throughout the area. Your own bodily electricity, like a fine and gentle brush, shoots out into the skin and underlying tissue.

Kirlian photography, a recent technological development, has produced graphic proof that the body itself is permeated and surrounded by a field of energy. (Kirlian photography is also called "high voltage photography".) What is clear from the research already done with this remarkable new technique is that the body's energy does not cease at the outer level of the skin. Energy surrounds the body itself, and is usually most intense around the head and hands. With the aid of your senses—that is, feeling the penetration of the heat (energy)—this energy can be made into a potent weapon against fat and waste accumulation.

When you are feeling the penetration of the energy from your hand, you are making your imaginative powers work for you. For the exercises to be fully effective, you must take the imaginative part of it seriously. What is becoming increasingly clear is that the way a person thinks, believes, and sees the world affects his or her physiological processes. For example, even the powerful malignancy of cancer can in some cases be brought to heel with the use of intensive visualization (or imaginative) techniques.

The Internal Exercises are expressions of the art of self- healing. The wisdom of the ancient Taoist sages makes it possible for these exercises to be unfailingly effective and safe, exceedingly simple to execute, and extremely efficient with human energy. The six exercises which are about to be described are among those arrived at through literally 6,000 years of observation and study of the natural principles of healing, and continual experimentation, selection, and perfection of techniques. It is only now that this ancient wisdom is becoming available to the West.

The Deer Exercise

The Deer Exercise is designed to generate and balance the secretions of the endocrine glands, particularly the sexual glands. It also strengthens the anal muscles. As a result, in the male the prostate is exercised and strengthened; and in the female, the vagina is exercised and strengthened.

In the Taoist definition of the immune system, the sexual glands form the base of the "immuno-glandular complex", the network of glands responsible for defending the body against disease-causing agents. These glands are, in ascending order from the base (sexual) glands, the adrenal glands, pancreas gland, thymus gland, thyroid gland, pituitary gland, and pineal gland. Their functions are supported by energy built-up within the sexual glands. A state of weakness or susceptibility to disease arises when one gland is for some reason deprived of energy to function. That is why energy built-up within the sexual gland is so important. When enough energy maintains the body's defenses, a constant state of health is ensured. And when diseases are prevented from disrupting the body's metabolic functions, the maintenance of proper weight will be ensured. The Deer Exercise serves this purpose.

The exercise is named after the deer because it appears to be constantly stimulating its anal area by wagging its tail. The activity was thought to strengthen the sexual glands and was adapted for human use.

MALE DEER EXERCISE

This exercise may be done standing, sitting, or lying down (on your back). Do this exercise in the morning upon rising, and before retiring at night.

1. Rub the palms of your hands together vigorously. This creates heat in your hands by bringing the energy of your body into your hands and palms.

2. With your right hand, cup your testicles so that your palm completely covers your testicles. (This exercise is best done naked.) Do not squeeze. Just a light pressure should be felt, as well as the heat from your hand going into your testicles.

3. Place the palm of your left hand on the area of your pubis, one inch below your navel.

4. Move your hand in clockwise or counterclockwise circles 81 times, with a slight pressure so that a gentle warmth begins to build in the area of your pubis.

5. Rub your hands together vigorously again.

6. Reverse the position of your hands (so that your left hand cups your testicles and your right hand is on your pubis). Repeat the circular rubbing motion in the opposite direction another 81 times.

7. Tighten the muscles around your anus. When done properly it will feel as if air is being drawn up into your rectum. Tighten as hard as you can and hold as long as you are able to comfortably do it.

8. Stop, and relax momentarily.

9. Repeat the anal contractions. Do this as many times as feels comfortable.

Note A: At first you may find you are only able to hold the sphincter muscles tight for several seconds. Please persist, and after several weeks you will be able to hold the muscles tight for quite a while without experiencing tiredness or strain. When done properly, a pleasant feeling will be felt to travel from the base of the anus, through the spinal column, to the top of the head. This is due to pressure being placed on the prostate gland as it is gently massaged by the action of tightening the anal muscles.

FEMALE DEER EXERCISE

This exercise can be done sitting on the floor or on a bed. Do the exercise in the morning upon rising, and at night before retiring.

1. Sit so that you can place the heel of one foot so that it presses into and up against the opening of your vagina. You will want a steady and fairly hard pressure so that the heel presses tightly against the clitoris. (If it is not possible to place your foot in this position, then use a fairly hard, round object such as a baseball.) You may experience a pleasant sensation due to the stimulation of the genital area and the subsequent release of sexual energy.

2. Rub your hands together vigorously. This creates heat in your hands by bringing the energy of your body into your palms and fingers.

3. Place your hands on your breasts so that you feel the heat from your hands enter into the skin.

4. Rub with your hands in an outward, circular motion. (Your right hand will turn counterclockwise, your left hand clockwise.)

5. Do this circular motion a minimum of 36 times and a maximum of 306 times.

6. Tighten the muscles of your vagina and anus as if you were trying to close both openings. When done properly it will feel as if air were being drawn up into your rectum and vagina. Hold these muscles tight for as long as you comfortably can.

7. Relax, and repeat the anal and vaginal contractions. Do this as many times as feels comfortable.

Note A: The first time you tighten these muscles, you may be able to do so only for a short time, but over time you will begin to build up the number of times you can do it, as well as the length of time you are able to hold the contractions.

Note B: The *outward* rubbing of the breasts (as in figure 3a.) is called *dispersion* and helps to prevent or cure lumps and cancer of the breasts. Reversing this (to an *inward* motion—so that the right hand circles clockwise and the left hand counterclockwise—is called *stimulation* , and its effect is to enlarge the breasts.

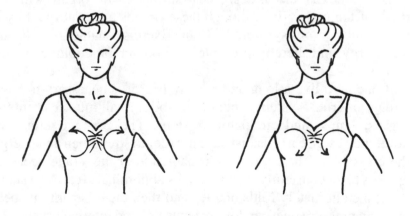

a. Dispersion   b. Stimulation

Figures 3a and 3b. The Female Deer Exercise.

Note C: Women should not perform the Deer Exercise during menstruation. At this time a natural imbalance of hormones occurs within the body and this exercise may tend to further stimulate the imbalance. Women should also not perform the Deer Exercise during pregnancy as the energy generated by the exercise, combined with the accompanying increased stimulation of the glands,might induce premature labor. Some women may find that their menstruation may stop as a result of practicing the Deer. This is not a cause for alarm, however, because the cessation of menstrual bleeding is a beneficial side effect of the exercise. When this occurs, needless bleeding and the consequent loss of nutrition may be avoided and used instead to strengthen the female system and balance the organs. The normal menstrual cycle will return upon ceasing to practice the Deer, with no detrimental side effects. Taoists refer to this phenomenon as "turning back the blood", since it may re-energize the entire body, especially the sexual organs.

The Crane Exercise

The Crane Exercise is designed to strengthen the organs within the trunk of the body. Even though these organs are controlled by the autonomic nervous system, the Crane Exercise enables us to balance the energy and thereby promote a smoother functioning of these organs.

If one is to live a long and healthy life, it is necessary to have a strong internal system, including abdominal muscles, internal organs, lungs, and circulatory system. The Crane Exercise was developed by an early Taoist sage in order to strengthen and energize these systems. The exercise was named after the crane because it appears to be constantly stimulating its abdominal area. As it stands, the crane alternately folds one leg and then the other into its belly, exerting pressure on its abdominal muscles and internal organs. This activity stimulates and strengthens the digestive, respiratory, and circulatory systems. The crane has an utterly different anatomical structure than does man; nevertheless, the principle upon which this characteristic movement is based is true and can be of use to us.

This exercise may be done standing, sitting, or lying down (on your back).

1. Rub the palms of your hands together vigorously. This creates heat in your hands and brings the energy of your body into your palms and fingers.

2. Place your hands, palms down, on your lower abdomen so that they lie on either side of your navel.

3. Inhale.

4. Begin to exhale slowly, pressing your hands down lightly so that your abdomen forms a hollow cavity. This gently forces the air out of your lower lungs. Imagine that every drop of air is leaving your lungs. (See figure 4a.)

5. After you have exhaled completely, slowly begin to inhale, extending your abdomen outward so it becomes like a balloon. Try not to allow your chest to expand—use only the muscles in your lower abdomen. (See figure 4b.)

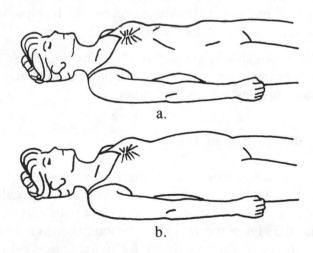

a.

b.

Figures 4a and 4b. The Crane Exercise.

6. One complete exhalation, followed by an inhalation constitutes one round of breathing. At first you will probably only be able to do two or three rounds of breathing at one sitting. Gradually increase the number until you have reached twelve rounds.

Note A: It is not necessary to force either the inhalation or the exhalation. With continued practice you will be able to extend and contract your abdomen quite easily while breathing very slowly. In the beginning your hands act as guides to help you learn the exercise. Once you have learned the breathing, it is not necessary to continue using your hands.

Note B: Once you have mastered the Crane exercise, you may combine the anal lock as described in the Deer Exercise with the Crane breathing. This will increase the strength of the exercise.

Note C: The best time to do the Crane Exercise is in the morning, if possible while facing the sun. Feel that as you inhale you bring the energy of the sun into your body, and that as you exhale all toxins and wastes are leaving your body.

Note D: When done before retiring at night, the Crane Exercise gives a gentle massage to the inner organs which helps calm the body, to relax us for proper sleep.

Note E: Women should not perform the Crane Exercise during pregnancy as the in and out motions of the abdomen may create unpleasant feelings within the abdomen.

SOLAR PLEXUS EXERCISE

The ancient Taoists believed that the vital organs in the torso were controlled by an "abdominal brain". Anatomically called solar plexus, this "brain" is a mass of nerve cells with nerves radiating outward like the rays of the sun. It can be found beneath the heart and behind the stomach. Responsibility for maintaining and balancing internal organ functions lies in the solar plexus. As a nervous center, it is where all nervous impulses generated by the abdominal organs concentrate for processing. When it becomes dysfunctional, the abdomen becomes distended. Dead cells, waste, and fatty tissues accumulate; and constipation, gastritis, ulcers, gastroenteritis, duodenal infection, diarrhea, and many other problems arise.

These conditions can be reversed or prevented by practicing the Solar Plexus Exercise, which protects, strengthens, and soothes the Solar Plexus. In a two-pronged attack against fatty accumulations and wastes, the exercise actively breaks up unwanted deposits while energizing the eliminatory process to flush the deposits of fat out of the body.

This exercise may be done standing or sitting. It can be done anywhere, anytime, and it can be included in your daily morning and evening exercise schedule.

1. While sitting or standing, place both hands on your stomach. Face front and inhale and feel the air expand your stomach.

2. Then exhale. As you exhale, use your hands to push your stomach in and up. As you execute these motions, turn your upper torso and head slowly toward your left side as far as possible and look to your left. Meanwhile twist your pelvis to the right.

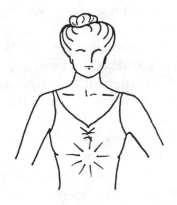

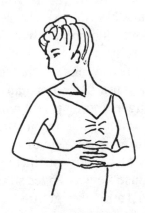

Figure 5.
The Solar Plexus.

Figure 6.
The Solar Plexus Exercise.

3. Inhale and bring your entire body back into alignment, facing front. As you do this, let your hands release your stomach slowly until they are resting gently on the skin surface.

4. Exhale again. But as you exhale, turn your upper torso and head slowly to the right side. Look to your right. Meanwhile push your stomach in and up again as you twist your pelvis to the left. (See figure 6.)

5. While inhaling, bring your body back into alignment, facing front. Repeat this exercise 4 to 36 times.

NOTE A: How many times you are able to do the exercise depends on the condition of your neck and shoulders. If you experience stiffness and pain at the neck and shoulders, do small repetitions until the condition clears. Then you may increase the repetitions in increments.

NOTE B: When you do the exercise, concentrate on the solar plexus area, which is located under the heart and behind the stomach. Try to feel heat (energy) penetrate into the solar plexus. The more you concentrate, the more benefits you gain from the exercise.

I lecture frequently on college campuses, and was one day in upstate New York. The dean of students, who was very overweight, looked much older than her years, and was in poor physical health generally. I suggested the exercise , demonstrating them for her. In just a few weeks she had lost five inches in her waist, hips, and thigh areas, and her color had come back to "normal". She became a younger, more vibrant woman, and is today head of one of the most important academic institutions in the nation.

Morgan was one of my most difficult cases. He came to me just after he had lost his influential job as head of a major airline; partly because he was under so much stress, he had become a compulsive eater, and was getting no exercise. He was also drinking large quantities of beer at the local bar. One day he heard that he had lost out on a major executive position with a Fortune 500 company—and it was only because of his sloppy appearance. Then he determined to stay faithfully with the exercise, did in fact slim down and firm up, and shortly thereafter was hired as president of a major food concern. I see him often, and he looks younger today than he did ten years ago.

STOMACH RUBBING EXERCISE

John, a bank president, was overweight, sluggish, and constipated. And, at age 55, he was almost ready to give up. His secretary urged him to try the simple Stomach Rubbing Exercise. By applying the exercise faithfully, he regularized his bowel movements, lost 40 pounds, and was filled with new energy.

An extremely overweight young woman of 29 came up to me after a lecture session to say that she feared she would never shed her excess inches—she was wearing a size 18 dress, and it was tight on her. She did not think she could stick with the Stomach Rubbing Exercise—so I tried to get her to see how easy it was. After trying the exercise, she realized that it was actually fun to do anyway, and within two weeks she noticed how loose her size 18 dress was becoming. So she stuck with the exercise, doing it daily no matter where she happened to be, and today she is down to size 11. When I first met her, she appeared to be in her 40's—and today she can casily pass for her very early 20's.

These are just a few of the results achieved by doing the Stomach Rubbing Exercise. It breaks up the fatty accumulations and deposits and passes them into the eliminatory system and out of the body. The superfluous areas of the stomach and abdomen are literally rubbed away.

This exercise should be done while lying down on your back. Do the exercise in the morning upon rising, and at night before retiring.

1. Begin by lying down flat on your back. Relax.

2. Put the palm of your hand on your navel. (If you are right-handed, use your right hand; if left-handed, use your left hand.) Then start to rub clockwise from the center—that is, from the

right to the left—first in small circles and then gradually expand the movement until the upper and lower limits of the stomach and abdomen are being rubbed (see figure 7a.)

3. When you have completed the first movement, then reverse it, rubbing counterclockwise in smaller and smaller circles until you are back to the center of the navel. You need not press down with any force. Apply a slight pressure as you rub slowly.

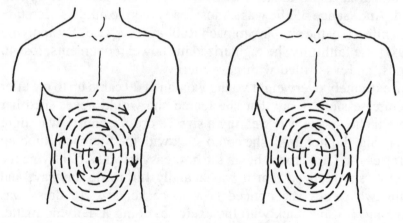

a. Clockwise Rubbing.   b. Counterclockwise Rubbing.

Figures 7a and 7b. The Stomach Rubbing Exercise.

4. Repeat this clockwise and counterclockwise motion as many times as you wish.

NOTE A: A brisker version of the Stomach Rubbing Exercise also exists. You may begin this exercise by rubbing the palms of the hands together vigorously and placing the hands, palms down, on the lower abdomen so that they lie on either side of the navel. Now begin to rub both sides of the abdomen briskly, following the pattern depicted in figure 8. Rub so that both hands meet near the navel on the downswing. Keep on rubbing until the friction heats up the abdominal tissues. You may repeat this exercise as many times as you wish. This version of the exercise brings more stimulation and energy to the abdomen than the regular version, so it can be used for debilitating diseases of the internal organs and peristaltic problems. It is especially good for trimming down the girth.

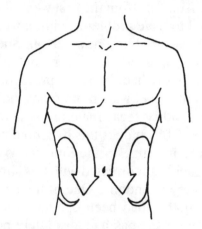

Figure 8. The Stomach Rubbing Exercise (brisker version).

NOTE B: For the exercise to be fully effective, concentrate on feeling heat (energy) penetrate into the area being massaged. The key is that warmth and energy. Relax. Let it burn off the excess fat. If your concentration wavers, begin again.

When you rub in a clockwise direction—which again, is from your right to your left in gradually widening circles—you are encouraging proper and easeful bowel movement. Quite often constipation is a symptom indicating that the large intestine is overfunctioning, and that toxins are accumulating. The large intestine is absorbing too much water from the waste matter as it passes through on its way to the rectum. This causes the waste matter to be compacted to the point where the normal peristaltic activity of the large intestine is not sufficient to expel the waste matter. Constipation results and fecal material that would normally have been passed on through the anus are stored in the body. The clockwise motion augments the peristaltic activity and slows down the water removal process to normal levels.

One young woman I taught this exercise to told me she had suffered from constipation most of her life. She was only 23 years old, but she had been suffering from constipation for 15 years. She had tried drugs, laxatives, and enemas. But nothing she did eliminated the problem. And yet, from the first week she began doing this exercise, she ceased to have problems with bowel movements. She felt, by her own admission, like a new person. She told me later that after three months of doing the exercise, her whole digestive system evened out and she never had the same problem again.

Rubbing in a counterclockwise motion has the opposite effect—that of helping to solidify fecal material as it passes through the intestine (see figure 7b). It does this by stimulating the passage of water from the large intestine to the kidneys. An extreme case of chronic diarrhea which was corrected with this simple technique was recently brought to my attention. One of my students told me that ten years ago his mother had been operated on for cancer of the colon. Since that time, she has had absolutely no control over her bowel movements. She could not even go out for fear she would suddenly find she had to use the bathroom and not have access to one. Her son taught her the stomach rubbing technique. She had tried every other remedy by that time and was ready for anything that held some promise of helping her. After a few days of practicing the exercise, her stools formed for the first time in ten years. Since then she has been able to normalize her life, and the problem has ceased to plague her.

Rubbing the abdomen in both the clockwise and counterclockwise directions will help stomach ulcers. One case demonstrating the exercise's efficaciousness is that of a ninety-six year old Chinese senator. He tackles his duties with more enthusiasm and energy than people one-fourth his age. He is also actively involved in many different activities. Yet he is never sick. His blood pressure, checked every morning by a government-appointed nurse, is always normal. When admirers ask him about his secret of youth, he tells them a story about a youthful experience. As a young man, he suffered from painful stomach ulcers, tuberculosis, and other diseases. When he served in the army, he sought medical help from doctors wherever he was stationed. Then one day, someone told him about a famous, aged healer who lived deep in the mountains. So he made an appointment to see the healer and struggled over the rocky terrain to see the healer. Upon reaching his destination, he greeted the healer, who was meditating, and began a monologue about himself and his problems. But the old man continued to meditate and seemed to ignore the visitor; he did not open his eyes or speak. Finally the healer uttered, "Go home and rub your stomach." Further questioning drew no replies, so the young man struggled home, disappointed at the simple remark. Back home, disappointment, exhaustion, and anger caused the ulcer to flare up again, and because he was left with no alternative, he reluctantly rubbed his stomach. Immediately the pain faded away. Encouraged, he began to rub his stomach faithfully. A few months later, the ulcer completely disappeared. Gradually the tuberculosis disappeared also, as his health improved daily. Thereafter for seventy years, he continually rubbed his stomach, after every meal and whenever he felt uncomfortable.

The first year I was invited to lecture at the University of Oslo in Norway, one of the subjects I dwelt on was the Stomach Rubbing Exercise. The following year, I was invited back to lecture before an overcrowded audience again. After lecture coordinator Dr. Bjorn Overbye introduced me and before I could speak, an old man in the audience interrupted me. After he asked for permission to speak, he told the audience to listen to me because whatever I said would be beneficial. Then he told everybody a story. He said that he attended my first lecture with a distended abdomen full of water because he had been suffering from terminal liver cancer. He was then in terrible pain. The doctors had given him only a few weeks to live. Every week he had to go to the hospital to have his abdomen pumped to remove the water. He was desperate to try anything when he attended the lecture. That night, after learning about the stomach rubbing technique, he went home and tried the exercise. To his astonishment, the pain immediately disappeared, and to his greater astonishment, water was later prevented from collecting in his stomach. One week later he went to see his doctor, who was also astonished. He then repeated his doctors words, "This is a miracle! I can't believe it! What did you do?" Smiling, he repeated his own words, "I didn't do anything. I just rubbed my stomach." He said that thereafter he faithfully rubbed his stomach, his liver did not bother him anymore, though it was still cancerous, and he was able to discontinue chemotherapy. Furthermore, he became "healthy", and was able to go back to work. When I returned to Norway in the third year, the man was still around.

Now, to summarize: the Stomach Rubbing Exercise has two principle components—the slow, circular rubbing motion, and the feeling of heat and energy filling the lower part of the body. The exercise should be performed twice a day (or more if you like) while lying on your back. The best times to do it are in the morning upon waking and then again just before you go to sleep. The rubbing motion begins at the navel and proceeds in ever larger circles in a clockwise direction (see fig. 7a). Once the whole area is covered, the motion is reversed, proceeding then in a counterclockwise direction (that is, from left to right) in gradually smaller circles until you find yourself back at the navel (see fig. 7b). All the while, you should be feeling heat or energy (in whatever way seems most congenial to you) warming the whole area. Try to see the blockages in your intestines breaking up and passing out of the body. Try to imagine the cells of fat actually melt away. You need not feel you must do it for a certain number of minutes for it to be effective. Performing the exercise for any length of time is better than not doing it at all! But do give it time to produce results for you and you will be gratified.

If you persist in this over time, you will reap other benefits as well. The Stomach Rubbing Exercise will improve the condition of your heart because you will have reduced its burden. The blood vessels will be gradually strengthened and your blood pressure will equalize. You will lose weight and inches and improve your digestion. You may very well notice an upswing in your level of vitality. Halitosis can be eliminated. All these processes are interlinked. And finally, the Stomach Rubbing Exercise acts as a natural sleeping draught. This is because when you rub the abdominal area, blood is drawn away from the head and brain. The usual mental chatter will be calmed, allowing you to drift into a restful sleep.

The Turtle Exercise

The Turtle Exercise is designed to aid a person in strengthening, relaxing, and eventually controlling the entire nervous system. It will reduce hunger in those who eat out of nervousness.

This exercise may be done standing or sitting.

1. Bring your chin down onto your chest. At the same time, stretch the top of your head upward. Inhale slowly as you do this. The back of your neck will feel a stretch upward and your shoulders will relax downward. (See figure 9a.)

2. Slowly bring the back of your skull as if to touch the back of your neck. Exhale slowly as you do this movement. Your chin will be pulled upward, and your throat will be slightly stretched. Also, your shoulders will be pulled upward on either side of your head as if you were trying to touch them to your ears. (See figure 9b.)

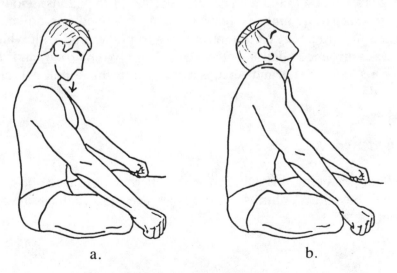

a.   b.

Figures 9a and 9b. The Turtle Exercise.

3. Repeat this cycle for a total of 12 times.

Note A: These two movements (or rather these two halves of one continuous movement) mimic the movements of the tortoise, as the animal pulls its head in and out of its shell. None of these movements need be forced, although it may take you a while before you become completely comfortable with the exercise.

Note B: The best time to perform the Turtle is just after rising in the morning, and just before retiring at night. You may also do it anytime you feel tension or tightness in your neck or upper back and shoulders.

This exercise, you will find with consistent practice, tightens, tones, and strengthens the muscles in your abdomen. Excess fat, water, and loose muscle will be eliminated, and a distended belly will shrink.

Mrs. Rosario ran a successful Italian restaurant in Chicago, and she nibbled at everything. Her husband was dead, and she was convinced that she would never attract the attention of any suitors at her age (she was 47) and with her weight (5'4", 175 pounds). Oddly, this stomach-flattening exercise not only slimmed her down, it seemed to help direct her interests away from the food with which she was surrounded daily. Today she is happily remarried, and she keeps her stomach flat and her hips trim by doing this simple exercise every day.

Weight Reduction Exercise

When practicing this exercise, remember never to force or push yourself beyond your limits. Acquire patience and steadiness in your practice.

PART ONE:

1. Stand against a wall so that your heels, buttocks, upper

back, and head are against the wall.

2. Inhaling through your nose, stretch your body upward, pulling your abdomen in as far as possible so your chest expands fully. Keep your arms by your sides. Your shoulders should feel as if they are expanding and pressing against the wall.

3. Keep your stomach muscles contracted for a moment.

4. Exhale as quickly as possible through your mouth. Blow the breath out fully and allow your stomach to extend as much as it can.

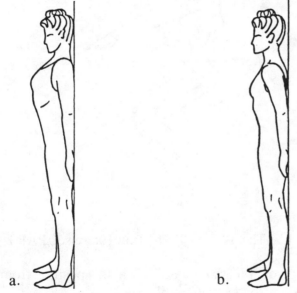

a.   b.

Figures 10a and 10b. The Weight Reduction Exercise, PART I.

5. Practice this inhale-exhale repetition 7 to 12 times.

You will find that with consistent practice, the muscles in your abdomen and belly will tighten and become toned and strengthened. Excess fat, water, and loose muscle will be eliminated, and your belly will shrink.

PART TWO:

1. Stand away from the wall and bring your heels off the floor so that you will be standing as high on your toes as possible.

2. Keeping your spine erect and straight, bend your knees slightly as if you were going to sit on a chair. Your arms will fall at a 45 degree angle from your body.

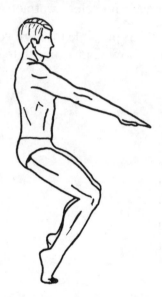

Figure 11. The Weight Reduction Exercise, PART II.

3. Keeping your breath regular, stay in this position from 10 to 20 seconds, or longer if possible.

NOTE: At first it will be impossible to keep your back straight and your heels up very far. With practice and practice, you will be able to get your heels perpendicular to the floor, your thighs parallel to the floor, and your back straight.

This exercise strengthens and tones the thighs, calves, and ankles. It makes the abdominal muscles strong, increases the circulation in the legs and body, and strengthens the back and the nerves in the body. It also stimulates the meridians of the bladder, gallbladder, and stomach. These meridians lie along the legs, and so it helps to reduce water retention and excessive weight and lowers the blood pressure.

Always practice both parts of the exercise at the same sitting as they balance and complement each other.

In addition to these exercises, there are other exercises designed to strengthen the limbs, muscles and bones. It usually takes three months to become proficient in these six basic Internal Exercises. The important point to make here, however, is that *self-healing*, which is the natural result of doing these exercises on a regular basis, is *guaranteed*.

PERSPIRATION

It is beneficial to do something which will cause you to perspire every day for 10 minutes. If you have access to a steam bath or sauna, that's excellent. If not, you can soak in the bathtub, with the temperature higher than your body's, for 10 minutes. DO NOT perspire for more than 10 minutes, or you will lose too much nutrition from the nutrients which escape in the liquid being eliminated through the pores. Keeping the perspiration period short also prevents you from becoming so thirsty that you end up drinking in more liquid than you perspire. If you must drink afterward, sip small quantities of liquid—enough to wet your tongue and satisfy your thirst.

Perspiration, as you may remember, will remove only water that is recently ingested. Perspiration alone can not dissolve cellulite deposits, because when cellulite accumulates, it is permanently retained and is difficult to remove. Cellulite deposits can only be broken up with heat, concentrated manipulation, and patience.

As you perspire, massage your body deeply with your fingers. Realize that you must squeeze the cellulite away with your bare hands. To do so, pick up the cellulite deposited skin between thumb and other fingers and knead the deposit thoroughly. This will help break up and dissolve the cellulite in the tissues. Release and pick up another deposit. Work on this area thoroughly. Using this method for ten minutes on one section of the body one day and on another section of the body another day, everyday, will gradually eliminate excess weight and improve skin and muscle tone. (Always keep in mind the limit on water intake.)

Success in cellulite elimination depends largely upon patience. Although you need only work on the deposits for 10 minutes a day, you must work on them daily for about three months (or less if the condition is less severe). If you try to hasten the slimming process, health problems may result, as they did for one lady. She probably thought that the ten-minute sessions were inadequate, so she stretched the ten-minute sessions into one-hour sessions. Unfortunately, she became very sick afterwards, as a result of breaking up too much cellulite and releasing too much of its toxins. Her body was unable to eliminate enough toxins in time to avoid toxic poisoning. Furthermore, by eliminating too much cellulite too quickly, she caused drastic changes in her body, changes her body could not readily adjust to. Cellulite bloats the tissues four to five times its original size. To accommodate its effects, the body must undergo many physiological changes over many years; it is completely different from what it used to be. Yanking the body back to its original state will harm its delicate functions and balance, and deny the skin a fair chance to regain its elasticity. So one must be patient and gentle in reversing the body's adjustments. Ten minutes daily is the rate that assures maximum cellulite elimination at the slightest risk to bodily health. After following this method faithfully and meticulously, many, many women were delighted with their extremely slim figures. So there need not be any hurry; a slim figure is guaranteed.

No ordinary diet will remove it for you. No cream or cosmetic will diminish it. Even if you fast, you will not take off a single ounce of it. And it is dangerous to your health. There is no doubt about that. You must act to remove it now.

A regime that claims to remove fat, without also removing cellulite, is tragically misleading-you. Your own mirror tells you the truth—if the cellulite remains, your body is not really becoming thin. You have not yet escaped the worst perils of being overweight.

ACUPRESSURE

These techniques use the pathways of vital energy (meridians) to calm and remove nervousness, stress and tension, and to decrease the appetite. At the same time they improve metabolism. Certain meridian points can be used:

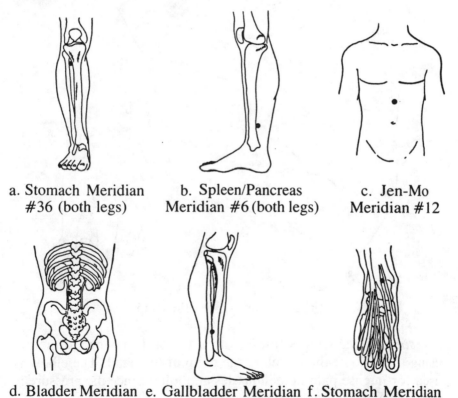

a. Stomach Meridian   b. Spleen/Pancreas   c. Jen-Mo
  #36 (both legs)   Meridian #6 (both legs)   Meridian #12

d. Bladder Meridian e. Gallbladder Meridian f. Stomach Meridian
 #23 (on both sides)   #38 (both legs)   #40 (both feet).

Figures 12a — 12f. Meridian Points.

All of these points can be used, but Stomach #36 must be used every time.

To apply pressure on these points, simply follow these indications.

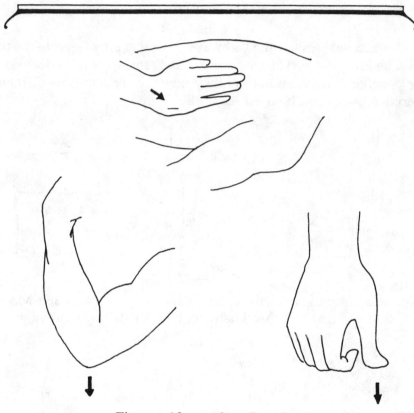

Figures 13a—13c. Pressing.

Pressing. Always press firmly with a forward, downward motion using the bulb of the thumb or the palm of the hand. The elbow is used for intense pain in the muscles and joints since the pressure is stronger and penetrates more deeply.

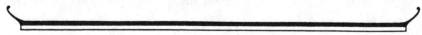

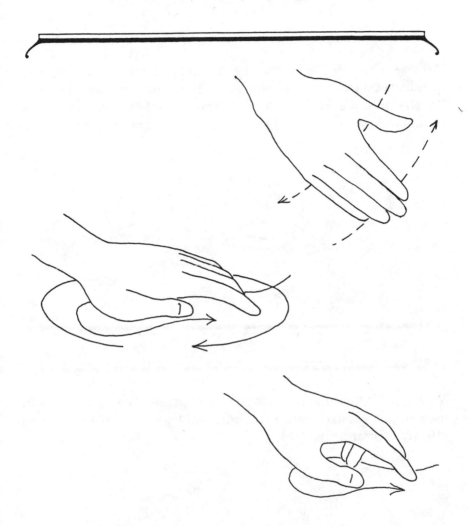

Figures 14a—14c. Soothing Stimulation.

Soothing Stimulation. Using the bulb of the thumb, the fingers, or the palm of the hand, massage with a light and rapid motion. The end result of this type of massage on painful areas of the body can be described as a soothing stimulation.

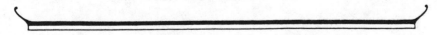

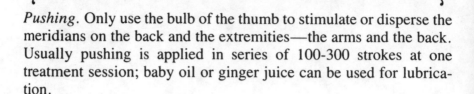

Pushing. Only use the bulb of the thumb to stimulate or disperse the meridians on the back and the extremities—the arms and the back. Usually pushing is applied in series of 100-300 strokes at one treatment session; baby oil or ginger juice can be used for lubrication.

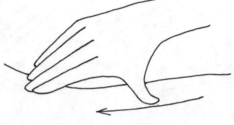

Figure 15. Pushing.

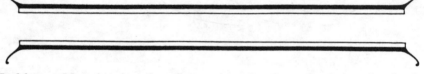

Rubbing. Use the thumbs, fingers, *and* palms. Both hands can be used simultaneously to rub the arms and legs. This method is very effective for arthritis.

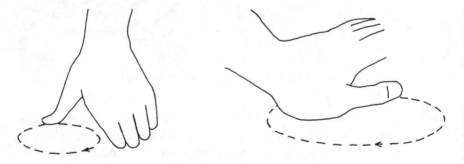

Figures 16a and 16b. Rubbing.

Acupuncture

Acupuncture should only be done by a qualified acupuncturist. Acupressure you may do yourself, or have a friend do to you.

CONSULT WITH YOUR DOCTOR

If you have health problems (see p. 43), you should see a physician before trying to take care of your weight problem yourself. In order to help these particular problems, certain Internal Exercises can be very helpful.

NUTRITION AND DIET

There are two basic proverbs to follow regarding diet:

a) *You are what you eat.* In other words what you put in your body becomes part of your body. If you put in healthy food, your body becomes healthy. If you put in garbage, your body becomes garbage. If you eat "cold" food you become cold. If you eat balanced food, you become balanced.

b) *You are what you metabolize.* What you eat is the basic foundation. But what you metabolize ultimately decides how that food will be used. If your body can digest and absorb what it needs, and eliminate what it does not need, your body will be healthy. If your body cannot take what it needs from the food you eat, or if it eliminates what it needs, or cannot eliminate what is toxic, your body will become weak, unhealthy, and eventually overweight.

According to the viewpoint of Taoists, a balanced diet is an essential pillar of good health. And that good health will support a life of longevity and happiness. The result of 6,000 years of experience, Taoism provides a complete and proven system to help people maintain healthy, well-balanced bodies.

Part V of this book contains 60 recipes for complete health and balanced nutrition. These recipes can be used in many, many combinations for breakfast, lunch, and dinner to provide an exciting and varied daily diet which you will never tire of.

PART III

4

Taoist Theories of Health and Physiology

One cannot understand the role that nutrition plays in weight control until the overall concept of health is understood from the Taoist viewpoint. This is because health and ideal weight are synonymous, and because diet is directly responsible for the state of one's health.

Health, in Taoist terms, is synonymous with balance. A truly well-balanced body—one in which all the organs and glands are functioning properly and regularly—is also a truly healthy body. Any imbalance in any of the body's functions is an indication of the absence of health. Imbalance equals weakness and/or disease.

Some outward signs of imbalance or weakness in the body associated with being overweight are heart problems, thyroid problems, shortness of breath, and susceptibility to infections. But there are other, possibly more hidden, symptoms or problems associated with unbalanced weight.

I must emphasize again that in order to understand this one must first explore the idea that the body is a self- supporting and self-regulating system, and that each body organ and function is dependent upon the functioning of all other organs, either directly or indirectly. The body is one whole, connected entity; it is not a series of fragmented parts hooked up together in an unrelated fashion.

Body function continues every second of the day from the cellular level on up.

THE FIVE ELEMENT THEORY

In order to make sense of how the different body functions and organs relate to and affect one another, Taoists devised the "Five Element Theory". They observed that there were five "elements" in the universe—water, fire, earth, metal, and wood—and that these five elements relate to each other in a way so as to stabilize the universe (and everything in it, including ourselves), even as it changes. That is, every movement in one direction is controlled by a movement in the opposite direction. Basically, there are two cycles—the Cycle of Generation and the Cycle of Degeneration or Control. All of the five elements are interrelated in both of these cycles. (See figures 17 and 18 on pages 88-89.)

Any one of our body's organs falls into one of the five categories of elements: metal represents the lung and large intestine, wood represents the liver and gallbladder, earth represents the spleen-pancreas and stomach, water represents the kidney and bladder, and fire represents the heart and small intestine.

THE FIVE TASTES

Since the Five Element Theory applies to every facet of existence, it also encompasses all types of food. In this case, the five elements are represented by the Five Tastes. Any food will fall into one of these five groups. Food is divided in this way because each group (taste) of food affects the organs it is related to within the Five Element Theory. For example, foods with a bitter taste will be guided to the heart, so bitter foods nourish the heart. The nutrients and vital energy in a bitter food will enable the heart to build more tissues, thereby strengthening itself and improving its function. Anyone who has drunk two or three cups of strong coffee within a brief period has experienced his heart "beat like crazy". Since coffee is bitter in taste, it directly affects the heart. Unfortunately it gives little or nothing in the way of nutritional help to the heart. It simply stimulates it to beat faster.

The following is a chart of the five elements along with their related Organs/Bowels, Superficial Organs, Organ Opening, and Taste.

Table I

Element	Taste	Organ/Bowel	Superficial Organ	Organ Opening
Metal	Spicy	Lung/Large Intestine	Skin	Nose
Wood	Sour	Liver/Gallbladder	Nerves	Eyes
Earth	Sweet	Spleen-Pancreas/ Stomach	Muscles	Mouth
Water	Salt	Kidney/Bladder	Bones	Ears
Fire	Bitter	Heart/Small Intestine	Blood Vessels	Tongue

In other words, you can say that spicy or piquant food is food for the lungs and large intestine. So cinnamon, pepper, chili, and curry are good for colds and coughs. In fact, these same spices are the basis for many home remedies for this type of illness.

Sour food is food for the liver. Apples, grapefruit, and something known in Chinese cooking as Yellow Flower are examples of sour foods.

Sweet food is food for the pancreas. String beans are considered good for the pancreas.

Salt is food for the kidneys. Salt stimulates the kidney and makes it work. Too much salt, however, overworks the kidney and weakens it. A weakened kidney, as in the case of people who retain water, needs to rest; it does not need more stimulation of the type it receives from diuretics.

Table II
The Five Tastes of Food

Sweet		Sour	Bitter	Salty	Spicy
Almonds	Peanuts	Beef	Artichokes	Beef	Anise
Beans	(raw)	Barbecue	Asparagus	(prepared)	Basil
Beets	Peas	Sauce	Avocados	Bones	Cayenne
Black Eye	Pecans	Breads	Bamboo	Butter	Pepper
Peas	Pies	Buttermilk	Shoots	Canned	Chili
Bran	Pudding	Chicken	Black	Foods	Curry
Brazil Nuts	Pumpkin	Collards	Fungus	Caviars	Dill
Cabbage	Rice	Fish	Bitter	Cheeses	Garlic
Cakes	Sherbet/	(Fresh-	Melon	Egg	Ginger
Candy	Sorbet	water)	Bock Choy	Fish	Leek
Canned	Snow Peas	Fruitjuices	Broccoli	(Saltwater)	Liquor
Fruits	Soft Drinks	(most)	Cauliflower	Frozen	Lung
Carrots	Sorghum	Fruit (raw)	Celery	Foods	(any type)
Cereals	Squash	Liver	Chard	Ham	Mint
Coconut	Starch	(any type)	Chinese	Kidneys	Mustard
Corn	String Beans	Mayonnaise	Mustard	(any type)	Onions
Cream	Sugar	Meats (red)	Chocolate	Olives	Oregano
Cucumber	Sunflower	Pickles	Cocoa	(pickled)	Parsley
Dried Fruit	Seeds	Rose Hips	Coffee	Margarine	Pepper
Eggplant	Sweet	Salad	Endive/	Processed	Rhubarb
Eggnog	Potatoes	Dressings	Escarole	Foods	Thyme
Fava Beans	Sweetened	Salami	Gelatin	(most)	Truffle
Honey	Fruit	Sausages	Green	Salt	Vanilla
Ice Cream	Syrup	Sour Cream	Vegetables	Seaweed	Wine
Jicama	Walnuts	Sprouts	Heart	Shellfish	
Kale	Wheat	Tartar	(any type)	Soy Sauce	
Kentucky		Sauce	Leeks	Tofu	
Wonder		Tomatoes	Mushrooms		
Beans		Turkey	Mustard		
Lettuce		Vinegar	Greens		
Milk		Yeast	Napa		
Milk		Yogurt	Cabbage		
Beverages			Rutabagas		
Molasses			Spirulina		
Oatmeal			Tea		
Pancreas			Turnips		
(any type)			Vegetables		
Pastry			(green)		

As said before, bitter food is food for the heart. However, there are very few bitter foods available in Western diets. Fortunately for our hearts, there *are* many bitter herbs—or Forgotten Foods—which are available.

(Some conflicts may be found within the list. If a food does not seem to belong where it is placed, it is because that food will change inside the human body.)

Table III
Five Tastes Balanced Diet

To maintain a balanced diet, according to the Theory of Five Tastes, over each twenty-four hour period food intake should be as follows:

SWEET	20%
SOUR	20%
BITTER	20%
SPICY	20%
SALTY	20%

Table IV
Excessive Sweet Taste Diet

If a person does not follow this dietary balance, illness and health problems will develop. For example, if a person's food intake produced these percentages:

SWEET	50%
SOUR	30%
SPICY	10%
BITTER	5%
SALTY	5%

the following health problems might occur: hypoglycemia, diabetes, heartburn, indigestion, constipation, water retention.

Table V
Excessive Sour and Salty Taste Diet

If the percentages were:

SWEET	20%
SOUR	30%
SPICY	10%
BITTER	10%
SALTY	35%

there is a strong likelihood of developing kidney weakness and disease, heart ailments, and high blood pressure.

The key criterion here is balance. If an organ is too weak, you cannot overstimulate the organ without making it weaker in the long run. For instance, too many apples a day (sour) would further fatigue a weak liver eventually, even if it is activated and appears stronger temporarily. In this case the Taoist science of nutrition would bring about an equilibrium within the body in order to deal more completely and delicately with the liver. According to the Five Element Theory, the five elements (as well as the organs they represent) support and control each other mutually, according to a pre-established order:

Water generates Wood
Wood generates Fire
Fire generates Earth
Earth generates Metal
Metal generates Water

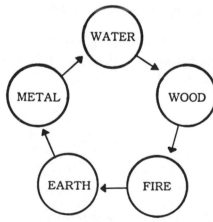

Figure 17.
Generating Cycle.

In this cycle, each element strengthens the successive one through a generative process, and each element becomes stronger and stronger along this wheel of creation.

Figure 18. Destructive Cycle.

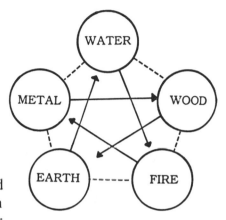

Water destroys or controls Fire
Fire destroys or controls Metal
Metal destroys or controls Wood
Wood destroys or controls Earth
Earth destroys or controls Water

In the destructive cycle, the elements mutually reduce the strength of each other and compensate for the generating process taking place in the generating cycle. These balancing equilibriums are used in Taoist healing and nutrition to ''tune up'' the function and health of individual body parts. For instance, by strengthening the kidney (water) you indirectly strengthen the liver (wood), as water generates wood according to the Five Element Theory. By calming or regulating over-functioning lungs (metal), you also ease the burden on the liver (wood), since metal controls or destroys wood. Thus, a weak liver can be brought to normality by tuning up the organs related to it. The applications of these interrelationships also apply to various levels in the body from the organs (the deepest) to the bowels (the superficial organs) to the organ openings (the most superficial), as shown in the previous table. For instance, someone with weak kidneys is prone to ear aches, ringing ears, and ear infections. Stronger lungs (metal) will strengthen the kidneys (water)—metal generates water—and will indirectly remove the susceptibility to earaches (see table I).

The key to stimulation and the nutritional provisions for tissue build-up of the various parts of the body is dictated by its taste, as explained before. This idea applies to *all* foods—the kind we buy at the grocery store as well as herbs.

ENERGY LEVEL OF FOOD

The regulation, or "tune up", of the body's general functions must also involve an understanding of the amount of energy supplied to the different body parts by the food eaten.

Table VI

Energy Level	Energy Characteristic	
Hot	Very energizing	
Warm	Mildly energizing	Yang
Neutral	Neither adds nor reduces energy	
Cool	Mildly energy reducing	
Cold	Very energy reducing	Yin

Cool or cold foods are "Yin". If the body is tense and congested, cool or cold foods can be used to release the blocked energy. As a rule, cold and cool foods such as fish should be cooked with a little bit of hot food to balance the energy, in order to prevent the loss of too much energy.

Below are listed some of our commonly eaten foods, which are categorized according to their hot, cold, warm, cool, or neutral energy characteristics.

Table VII

Cold	Cool	Neutral	Warm	Hot
Celery	Algae	Eggs	Beans	Chili
Freshwater	(Spirulina)	Grains	Beef	Cinnamon
Fish	Butter	Tea	Coffee	Garlic
Shellfish	Dairy Products	Tofu	Poultry	Ginger
	Fruit (most)		Root	Lamb
	Green Vegetables		Vegetables	Pepper
	Mushrooms		Vegetable	Wild Game
	Oils		Flowers	
	Pork			
	Processed or			
	Frozen Foods			
	Seafood			
	Sprouts			
	Sugar			

This intrinsic balance at the organ level should also be tied in with the body's overall functions, i.e., according to the Five Element Theory. A liver (wood) weakened by excess alcohol intake (and therefore having a low energy level) will break the stand-off or controlling balance it has with the stomach (earth). Being free from control, the stomach will then begin to overwork. Part of this over-functioning results in an excess of acidic secretions by the stomach and the creation of heartburn sensations.

The Taoist energy theory applied to nutrition unveils a whole dimension neglected in Western dietetic science. For example, lamb, which is hot, will contribute additional energy, while pork, which cool, will reduce that energy level. (Pork is helpful in times of congestion, but it has an adverse effect in the case of weakness.)

ENERGY BALANCE OF FOOD

The energy or vital force must be balanced between the organs for smooth functioning and perfect digestion and metabolism. Each food provides its own level of energy, and the energy intake as a whole must match the body's needs and compensate for the imbalances which may already exist in the body.

The energy referred to here is the vital force which keeps our blood circulating and our organs functioning. Without that energy our body would be like a perfect machine without the force or fuel to make it run. This energy represents the essence of life, and contributes to the natural processes of bodily growth, repair, and response to disease and infection. This energy should not be confused with the calories identified in medical science. The latter represents the fuel consumed in muscular efforts.

Each food has a different energy level that ranges from "cold" to "hot". A food with warm or hot energy will bring vital energy to the organ affected, according to the corresponding taste. A food with a cool or cold energy will reduce the vital energy level of the organ affected, according to the corresponding taste (see table VI). A weak organ (i.e., one lacking energy) needs food with warm or hot energy in order to be revitalized. It is the opposite with an inflamed organ which needs to be fed cool or cold food to reduce the inflammation (energy level). Neutral food neither adds nor drains energy from the body.

Hot and warm foods are considered to be "Yang", that is, positive and energizing. Hot foods are too energizing to eat a great deal of. Ginger, for example, is a very "Yang" food, and while safe in small quantities and mixed with other balancing foods, it can be very harmful if used in large quantities or by itself.

If you are weak, you need warm food. Many people practicing a vegetarian diet will add fish to their regimen hoping that the additional protein will give their overall energy level a boost. Instead, the fish, which is cool, weakens or lowers their energy level even further, by taking even more energy out of their bodies.

Similarly, high calorie foods may deplete the level of vital energy in the body. For instance, sugar, while high in calories, also has a cool energy level. Excessive consumption of sugar will deplete the vital energy lodged in the pancreas (related to the sweet taste by the Five Element Theory) and weaken its function. The weak pancreas will then "leak" excessive insulin into the blood and neutralize the blood sugar.

SEASONAL CONCEPT OF EATING

There may be some teachings which insist upon the so called seasonal concept of eating. In those teachings, the elements and associated tastes are assigned to each and every month of the four seasons, causing one taste to be primarily associated with one season. That means a person has to eat foods of primarily one taste for several months—a practice true Taoists completely avoid. There is a warning against such unbalanced methods of eating in chapter 27 of the *Nei Ching*, Yellow Emperor's book of Internal Medicine. It is stated that overuse of any of the five tastes will lead to disaster. Eating too much sour foods over an extended period of time over-stimulates and damages the liver, gallbladder, and nervous system. Similar abuse of spicy foods weakens the lungs, large intestines, and skin. Overeating salty foods for a lengthy period of time weakens the kidneys, bladder, and bones. Likewise, overuse of sweet foods weakens the spleen-pancreas, stomach, and muscles. Finally, over-eating bitter foods weakens the heart, small intestines, and blood vessels.

If one still were to apply the seasonal concept of eating, then one must also apply yearly, daily, even hourly concepts of eating. According to the Five Element Theory, the elements are also assigned to yearly, daily, and hourly portions of time, besides the monthly (seasonal) portion of time. So one simply can not embrace one concept and forget the rest. But applying all the concepts of eating will result in great confusion, as described in the following paragraphs. Either way one loses. That is why true Taoists do not teach such concepts of eating.

The yearly, monthly (seasonal), daily, and hourly concepts of eating are outlined in the following table:

Table VIII

The Elements in Relation to the
Hours, Days, Months, Seasons, and Years.

ELEMENT	WOOD		EARTH	FIRE		EARTH	METAL		EARTH	WATER		EARTH
YEAR	1986	1987	1988	1989	1990	1991	1992	1993	1994	1995	1996	1997
SEASON	SPRING			SUMMER			AUTUMN			WINTER		
MONTH	Feb.	Mar.	Apr.	May	Jun.	Jul.	Aug.	Sep.	Oct.	Nov.	Dec.	Jan.
DAY	Jan. 5, 1987	Jan. 6, 1987	Jan. 7, 1987	Jan. 8, 1987	Jan. 9, 1987	Jan. 10, 1987	Jan. 11, 1987	Jan. 12, 1987	Jan. 13, 1987	Jan. 14, 1987	Jan. 15, 1987	Jan. 16, 1987
HOUR	3-5 a.m.	5-7 a.m.	7-9 a.m.	9-11 p.m.	11-1 p.m.	1-3 p.m.	3-5 p.m.	5-7 p.m.	7-9 p.m.	9-11 p.m.	11-1 a.m.	1-3 a.m.

According to the above table, 1986 and 1987 are wood (or sour) years; 1988, an earth (or sweet) year; 1989 and 1990, fire (or piquant) years; 1991, an earth (or sweet) year; 1992 and 1993, metal (or spicy) years; 1994, an earth (or sweet) year; 1995 and 1996, water (or salty) years; 1997, an earth (or sweet) year; 1998 and 1999, wood (or sour) years—the twelve-year cycle begins again. According to the above table, twelve months complete a cycle, the next twelve another cycle, and so on. Also, a cycle is completed every twelve days and every twelve hours. If we abandoned our common sense and mechanically followed the pattern of eating described above, we would be eating sour foods for four hours, then sweet foods for two, followed by bitter foods for four hours, and so on throughout the day. We would also be eating foods of only one taste for 48 hours, followed by foods of another taste for 24 hours, and so on. We would also be eating foods of one taste for one or two months. And we would be eating foods of one taste for a maximum of two years. How we are going to determine what foods to eat when the element of the hour clashes with the element of the day, when the element of the day clashes with that of the month, when the element of the month clashes with that of the year, no one knows. How our organs are going to handle so much salt, spice, etc. all at once, no one knows either. Beginning with the Yellow Emperor, all true Taoists regarded such concepts of eating as completely illogical, unfeasible, and above all unbalanced and harmful.

FORGOTTEN FOODS

It is important to have a balanced diet, as already defined, in order to maintain good health, or not to aggravate an existing bodily imbalance. However, some imbalances, created by serious disease (such as hepatitis) or serious abuse cannot be corrected by the food encountered in our regular food markets, despite use of the Taoist knowledge of common diet. For example, an imbalance resulting from damage to the liver tissues can only be perfectly reversed through the implementation of foods or herbs called "Forgotten Foods". These foods, such as the bupleurum tree for the healing of the liver, have been neglected down through the centuries as our ancestors gradually limited their diet to foods of pleasing taste or easy commercialization. The science of Forgotten Foods— Herbology—represents a separate and complex knowledge of its own and is not explained here because of its immensity.

PH BALANCE OF FOOD

When people hear the term "balanced diet", they think of the generally accepted idea of eating food belonging to all of the "Basic Four Food Groups" so often discussed by Western nutritionists.
There is another aspect of "balance" in the diet which is essential

to our health. This balance has to do with the levels of acid and alkaline in the food we eat. If the food in our stomachs is too acid or too alkaline, it is not properly assimilated by our bodies. In addition, food with poor pH (acid-alkaline) balance is digested too slowly, giving it a chance to decompose in our digestive tract. When this happens, this decomposing food becomes a welcome home for germs and parasites which enter our bodies through our food. The pH balance in the stomach keeps germs away while the body metabolizes the food. If the pH balance is missing, the food is corrupted immediately by the microorganisms in the food and body. The body, instead of benefiting from the nutrients in the food, absorbs the poisons resulting from the corruption. (If one ever goes to the back door of any restaurant, one will find food corrupting in garbage cans. Not long ago, this food was served to customers. So the only thing separating the front and back of the restaurant is a wall and a few hours' time.) We would not purposely eat garbage because we know we would become sick from ingesting its poisons. Yet, we do eat garbage every time we eat without a thought for pH balance. (A telltale sign of food corruption in the stomach is bad breath.)

If our food is balanced, it passes quickly and efficiently through our digestive tract, and the waste passes out of our bodies in the form of stools. This all happens before the food has an opportunity to become a home for unwanted organisms.

The typical American diet contains an abundance of acid foods and very little alkaline foods, which explains the success of antacid tablets (which are alkaline) in this country. When consumed, these alkaline pills neutralize the acid in the stomach. This brings temporary relief (just as the television commercials say). What they neglect to say is the stomach *needs* acid in order to digest our food. Neutralizing our stomach acid with pills results in food remaining in our stomach. Eventually the stomach must produce more acid in order to digest it; this produces heartburn, and we again have to take antacid pills. Thus a cycle is established of alternating between heartburn and the ingestion of antacid pills.

A look at a typical menu will give you a clearer idea of just how much acid is in our diet:

Table IX

Acid	Alkaline
1. Pre-dinner cocktail, tea or fruit juice (all alcohol is acid)	1. Small portion of green vegetables
2. Soup (if tomato based)	2. Baked potato
3. Bread (or croutons)	
4. Salad dressing	
5. Meat, fish, or cheese entree	
6. Wine	
7. Dessert	
8. Coffee, tea, or juice	

Acid foods outweigh alkaline foods by 8 to 2! Not only that, but to properly balance the servings of meat and vegetables, you should eat an equal amount of vegetables and meat, so your meal should consist of 50% meat and 50% vegetables. The only way to be sure of getting the right pH balance in your meals is to be aware of what you need, and to plan your meals accordingly.

Table X

Acid/Alkaline Balance of Foods.

The following chart shows which foods are acid and which are alkaline in theory. (In some cases, these foods may trigger a response in the stomach that completely negates their effects. For example, some alkaline foods may cause the stomach to secrete more acids. Once in the stomach that food is actually acidic.)

Acid		Alkaline
Alcohol (all)	Fish	Cooked Vegetables
Bread (or Croutons)	Fruit Juices	Grains (including Rice)
Cheese	Meat	Green Vegetables
Coffee	Salad Dressings	Potatoes (baked or boiled)
Deep Fried Foods (all)	Soups (tomato based)	Sprouts
Desserts	Tea	

NUTRITIONAL BALANCE

It is said that we should have nutritionally "balanced" meals, such and such an amount each day of proteins, vitamins, minerals, and other "foods". If you ask me whether or not you need these, my reply would be "What are vitamins? What are minerals? What are proteins?" And "How much knowledge do we really have about them?"

The point is that "proteins", "vitamins", and "minerals" are just terms developed by scientists who study foods in order to determine what kind of effective composition they contain. Each time scientists discover new components, they invent new names to "explain" what these components are. They also attempt to explain a food by the components they have isolated within that food. For example, scientists have found Vitamins A, C, Fructose, Pectin, and Laetrile in apples. So they say an apple will supply these nutritional components. Or, worse yet, they say if you take these components individually, you can substitute them for an apple.

Most people know that an apple is not only composed of Vitamin A, C, Fructose, Pectin, and Laetrile. Most scientists recognize that there are probably two thousand additional components in an apple which are still unnamed at this time. When we eat an apple, vitamin A is released from the apple by an enzyme in the intestinal wall and is absorbed along with the two thousand or so released components. All at once, balanced nutrition is easily obtained. But if we separated those components from the apple and took them by themselves, and then neglected to eat the real apple, we would be misusing our scientific knowledge. We shortchange ourselves of full nutrition when we take natural or synthetic vitamins.

You should also know that whenever you take *synthetic* vitamin tablets, you are taking a risk. Most people do not know that most of the synthetic vitamin supplements are not derived from "regular" sources. Vitamin C, for example, is not separated from oranges and then formed into tablets. Instead it is synthesized from sugar in an inexpensive, four-step process involving enzymes and chemicals.

98

Traces of the chemicals used in, or resulting from, vitamin synthesis may remain in the end-product. Because some chemicals can be toxic, the end-product can also be toxic. We have no idea what chemical reactions arise when the incoming chemical compounds meet the intestinal secretions, which are also chemicals. Also, most of us have no way of determining how much supplements our bodies need. Forcing large amounts of any vitamin on our bodies can lead to trouble. For example, long-continued large doses of vitamin A can cause decalcification of bones, bone swellings, headaches, diarrhea, nausea, etc. These problems can be avoided if the body is given a chance to isolate and absorb what it needs for itself.

I respect the known scientific knowledge and I think it is valuable, but it is incomplete, and I do not feel we should be overly attached to or be dependent on the theories of an area that is not yet fully known. Food *components* are not sufficient for good health. We should eat whole foods, in as natural a state as possible. There have been instances of hunger strikers who have been given "perfectly balanced nutrition" injections—and then died from malnutrition. Their bodies could not absorb or utilize the "solid" scientific principles of nutrition. A similar thing happens when you take a vitamin B tablet; it is rejected instead of being absorbed like coffee or other naturally occurring foods. We know that when we drink great amounts of black coffee something entirely unlike coffee (urine) is excreted two hours later. That is because coffee undergoes many chemical changes when it goes through the many intestinal departments, mixes with the secretions of each, and gets broken down, absorbed and filtered. Well this does not happen when we take a vitamin B tablet. As a tablet, before it is swallowed, vitamin B has a distinctive yellow color and odor. After it is swallowed and passed through the entire digestive process, the vitamin emerges two hours later as chemically unchanged as a new tablet—the urine smells and looks strongly like liquid vitamin B. The body does not absorb or utilize the vitamin at all. If we were to inject the vitamin into the bloodstream, we would get the same results. Often, vitamin B is ejected out of the pores of the skin with the perspiration, causing an entire room to be filled with its odor. Even if vitamin B were chelated (predigested) or formed into time-released tablets, the body would still reject the vitamin completely. None of these problems would be experienced if vitamin B "pills" such as beans, vegetables, etc. were eaten. Vitamin B is found in high concentrations in these foods, yet when these foods are eaten, the distinctive color or odor is never detected.

There is still a great deal to understand about the effectiveness of vitamin supplements. There are those who swear vitamin C cures cancer, prevents colds, etc., and there are those who think otherwise. In the most recent scientific research done on vitamin C, no evidence whatsoever was found to support the claim that vitamin C cures cancer. This announcement was made by research teams at both Stanford University and Harvard University. Not only does vitamin C fail against cancer, but it also aggravates stomach ulcers, causes kidney stones and stomach over-acidity, etc., if it is over-used. Almost daily, new claims emerge about the curative properties of vitamins and new facts emerge to disprove them.

The conclusion is that this field of knowledge is just too young to rely on, and it is likely to remain so in the near future. It is better to rely on 5,000 year old wisdom teachings that have been proven effective time and again. After all, no matter how smart a twenty-year old boy is, he can not be smarter than a 5,000 year old wise man. This is not to say that science will never achieve a complete under-standing of what a true "nutritional balance" is—it will several hundreds or thousands of years from now. But that need not deter you. Because if you follow the 5,000 year old principles of this book you will be eating whole, healthy foods—not vitamins, proteins, and minerals. You will realize that the old saying was not "Vitamin A, C, Fructose, Pectin, and Laetrile a day keeps the doctor away". It was "an apple a day keeps the doctor away". And you will be eating the whole apple, or whatever food it may be. You will be secure in the knowledge that every component of that food—whether it be called vitamin, protein, mineral, or whatever—is in just the right amounts, and in perfect proportion and balance to all other compo-nents of that food. Indeed it is a law of nature that were they not in balance, it would not be possible for that food to even exist, for balance is a basic foundation of the reality of nature.

5

How to Use the Given Information

This weight loss book is much more than the usual diet book. It presents an entire theory of nutrition based on principles which have been proven for over 6,000 years. And it offers simple techniques and exercises based on these theories. These techniques and exercises have been developed, refined, and perfected over many, many centuries. The ancient lineage of Taoist teachers and researchers were and are very practical. If a technique did not work, it was discarded. If another one was developed which worked better than an earlier one, it replaced it. The end result is the knowledge in this book: solid, practical information which will help you control your weight, improve your health, and prevent disease and other physiological disorders. Of course it is you who must ultimately take responsibility for your own health. This book will give you the tools and information you need to do this. In the simplest and most enjoyable way possible. You will be amazed at the results.

1. Read the book through—slowly. You have probably already played the "diet game" for years, so there is no need to rush. Now you have finally found something that will work. And this book will give you the general overview you need to really understand why the results you will get are possible.

2. Re-read any section you care to repeat. There may be some sections that escape total absorption on the first examination.

3. Skim over the *Eight Causes of Weight Problems* again. Your main concern is how to get rid of excess weight. But this section will give you a good understanding of why you are where you are. And it may give you a few hints for helpful changes you can make in your lifestyle.

4. Check with your physician if you have any doubts about making changes in your diet or physical activities.

5. Begin restricting your liquid intake to just under 6 cups of fluids a day. I cannot stress this too much. Even if you were to throw the book away right now, and followed this one technique only, you would experience dramatic improvement in your body over a few weeks.

6. Begin to do, whenever possible, the Stomach Rub. It is a deceptively simple exercise which can produce remarkable results. The same applies to the other figure-slimming exercises.

7. Skim over the sections on *Taoist Theories of Health and Physiology* and the *Dietary Do's and Don't's*. This will refresh your memory on the basic theory and rules of good nutrition.

8. Begin using the recipes in this book. Start with just one meal a day (preferably but not necessarily breakfast), continuing with your normal diet for the other two meals.

9. Gradually expand your use of the recipes until you are using them for all meals.

10. As you begin to eat and enjoy the nutritious and delicious meals described in this book, begin also to do the Internal Exercises. Start with the Deer Exercise. When you feel completely confident with that, begin to include the Crane Exercise. Then later, add the Turtle Exercise.

11. After you have reduced your liquid intake for a while, begin to make sure that each day you experience 10 minutes of

perspiration. This will help you to avoid water retention and to eliminate toxins. During these 10 minutes each day, do a deep manipulative massage of any part of your body which has cellulite deposits. This combination of massage and perspiration is the *only* way you can truly get rid of your unwanted cellulite.

12. Enjoy your new healthy body! It is a gift from God—and you deserve it!

Several years ago I spoke to a group of overweight wives of physicians. After my talk, one young woman turned to me and said, "Dr. Chang, I don't think my marriage is going to last. I love my husband, and he loves me, but I'm more than pleasingly plump. What can I do?" Well, she was about 5'9'', and weighed about 210 pounds. But I noticed that her weight was mostly in her mid-sections, front and back. I suggested the exercise. Several weeks later the young wife called me to say that her figure was "straightening out". I saw the couple quite recently, and she is nicely proportioned. Her husband now paid her close attention (as did all other men in her presence), and they were obviously quite happy.

Although I wouldn't recommend that a person continue to eat and drink excessively, let me give you an example of a man who did just that and still managed to lose inches. Paul C. is an acquaintance of mine who attended one of my lectures in Phoenix, Arizona. Now, this man was nothing short of obese, and he was still gaining weight. He told me that eating was his chief pleasure in life and he didn't see that he would be willing to give it up. "But is there a way for me to lose this stomach?" he asked me, pointing to his distended belly. Mr. C. was obviously a "hard case", but I recommended that he do the exercise. I got a call from him a month later, and he told me gleefully that he had already lost three notches on his belt! He continued to lose weight until he had stabilized into a normal range, but he still shows his friends his old belt.

Martha M.'s severe pain was diagnosed as a case of arthritis and other unknown reasons. The pain she suffered was so severe that she couldn't get up without assistance after someone helped her to sit down. Twenty-five doctors of an university medical center were involved in treating and researching her affliction for eight months. Finally two people carried her to my office. After obtaining her history, this diet program and certain exercises were suggested. And in four weeks, she came to see me by herself. She had only a cane to support her. After another four weeks she came again, this time without a cane.

Kirk D.:

I'm sixty-three years old. Two years of my life were spent in agony. I had a stroke and the entire left side of my body was paralyzed. After I followed Dr. Chang's instructions, I was able to button my own shirt in two weeks! After six weeks I was able to attend a football game on my own.

6

Dietary
Do's and Don't's

There are a number of dietary do's and don't's which are necessary to follow if we are to maintain a balance in the functioning of our bodies.

BODY SIGNALS

DO listen to your body and pay attention to its signals. Each person has a different system and reacts differently to each individual food. If you notice signs of mucus, pimples, diarrhea, or constipation after the consumption of certain foods, this is an indication that your system cannot assimilate the food properly, and that the food is irritating or poisoning your body in some way. This type of condition is commonly called food allergy. If a certain food affects you in one or more of these ways, avoid it.

CHOLESTEROL

Cholesterol is both useful and harmful to the body, according to the latest scientific studies. On one hand it is needed to synthesize vitamin D, hormones, etc.; on the other hand it can cause heart disease. Therefore, restricting oneself to low cholesterol or cholesterol-free foods to avoid heart disease is not the safest or healthiest solution. For example, according to Taoist experience, a restricted vegetarian diet can cause malformations, due to unavoidable deficiencies. The real problem is the combination of cholesterol and saturated fat. These two units, when combined, magnify each other's harmful aspects, and become the greatest enemies of the cardiovascular system. A lethal combination, for example, can be butter and shrimp.

CHRYSANTHEMUM FLOWERS

DO make a tea out of chrysanthemum flowers or drink teas made with these flowers.

A recent study proved that chrysanthemum flowers possessed potent cholesterol-reducing properties. In this study, two groups of mice were used: I and II. Group I was further divided into groups A and B; group II, C and D. Group A was given a high fat, high cholesterol diet. So was group B, except it had chrysanthemum flowers incorporated into its diet. Group C was given a low fat, low cholesterol diet. So was group D, except it also had chrysanthemum flowers added to its diet. The ingredients and amounts of the food given to all four subgroups were basically the same. Later, it was found that the blood cholesterol levels of group B were lower than those of groups A *and* C. So low, in fact, that they approximated those of group D. Of course the blood cholesterol levels of group A exceeded those of every other group. Chrysanthemum flowers were able to prevent high blood cholesterol levels in mice, even if their diets were high in fat and cholesterol.

This property of the chrysanthemum flower has been known to work for humans for thousands of years, and is only now coming to light. Still shrouded in secrecy, but known for thousands of years, are these properties: brain cell purification, hormone adjustment, and improvement of digestion and absorption. Chrysanthemum flowers also purifies the skin and improves its texture.

CRAVINGS

Food cravings indicate an imbalance in the body which can lead to food allergy. If you crave a particular food, this is an indication that your body has already had too much of it. Try to leave it alone—your body really does not need more of what it craves. Giving in to the craving can only lead to health problems in the long run.

Please note that we say DO listen to *certain things*—gas, indigestion, etc.—but NOT to *cravings* of any kind, whether they be sugar, water, meats, or whatever.

DIVERSITY

DO eat a diversity of foods. In so doing, you will satisfy your appetite in a way that cannot be done with limited eating habits. Your appetite will normalize itself and any desire to binge or overeat will dissipate.

Also, by eating a variety of foods—that is, foods representing all of the Five Tastes—your body will receive the balanced nutrition and energy it needs to function well. In addition, if you avoid a particular food, your body will suffer from some kind of shortage. In the long run, it will reject that particular food if it is ever eaten again, because it is not used to or estranged from the chemical elements in the food. This can lead to atrophy in some organs and many related problems.

EATING SCHEDULE

Again, DO eat on time. And DO eat when you are in a peaceful, loving state of mind. Eating when you are angry can have harmful effects on your well-being, because when you are angry the liver releases real poisons into your system.

DO NOT eat when you are extremely tired. There will be a lack of energy to digest food, and eating will result in undigested food and the resulting putrefaction and food poisoning. For this reason DO NOT eat immediately after sexual intercourse. Nor should you eat immediately before intercourse, for the same reason. Speaking of sex, if you engage in oral sex you should not consume semen if you are interested in losing weight. Semen, although small in quantity, is tremendously nutritious and could negate the efforts you make to lose weight.

FASTING

DO NOT fast, because fasting can atrophy the entire body. Many cases show that after fasting for a long period of time, people are not able to digest *any* food. The final result is death.

The universe is the macrocosm, the body is the microcosm. In other words, the human body represents all the elements of the universe. So we should eat a diversity of all universal substances. God intended it that way. He gave us the different flavors of food for our mental and spiritual pleasure, and for our physical needs. We need to nourish all three parts of ourselves—the mental, the spiritual, and the physical.

FATS

Taoists recognize the life-sustaining qualities of food *and* the deleterious qualities of food. Certain food components are capable of causing health problems and deadly diseases. This is especially true of fats, which, according to the Yellow Emperor, is the greatest dietary enemy of human beings. Now this 5,000 year old teaching is substantiated by American Institute for Cancer Research reports. According to scientific studies done on unsaturated and saturated fats, the risks of cancer and heart disease were lowered by decreased consumption of fats. The dietary guideline for lowering cancer risk is given below:

Table XI

Dietary Cancer Risk

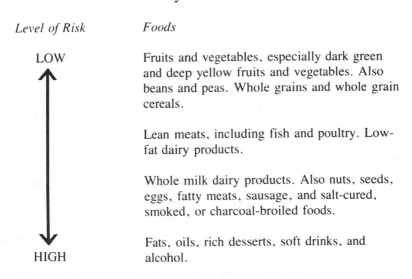

Level of Risk	*Foods*
LOW	Fruits and vegetables, especially dark green and deep yellow fruits and vegetables. Also beans and peas. Whole grains and whole grain cereals.
	Lean meats, including fish and poultry. Low-fat dairy products.
	Whole milk dairy products. Also nuts, seeds, eggs, fatty meats, sausage, and salt-cured, smoked, or charcoal-broiled foods.
HIGH	Fats, oils, rich desserts, soft drinks, and alcohol.

FIBER

DO include fiber in your diet. It is essential for the health of the large intestine. To function properly, the large intestine has to be filled up firmly, like a sausage, on a regular basis. The large intestine is very soft, and without anything to fill it, it shrinks, and the sides of the intestinal wall rub against each other, which can lead to ulcerations of the colon. This condition can gradually lead to cancer of the colon, as dirty waste deposits build up there, aggravating the condition further. Also, lack of fiber can be the cause of both chronic diarrhea and chronic constipation, which can lead to cancer because of chronic inflammation in the colon area.

Over one thousand years ago, the Chinese recognized the importance of fiber and decided that nothing in their daily diet included enough of it. That is why they added bamboo shoots to their diet. Today, bamboo shoots remain the best source of fiber, and can be found in most Chinese recipes.

Bamboo shoots are good for both chronic diarrhea and chronic constipation. I once treated a woman who had suffered from alternating constipation and diarrhea for twenty years through improper eating habits and the use of laxatives. I advised her to include bamboo shoots in her diet, to include as much as possible in her soups, salads, and other foods. The results were practically immediate, and she felt better than she had felt in twenty years. "What's in those bamboo shoots?" she asked. "Nothing," I replied. "They just fill up your intestines so they can work!" Bamboo shoots have no specific nutritional value—no vitamins, minerals, proteins, or acids.

Carrots are also a good source of fiber. However, since the nutrients of *raw* carrots or carrot juice are not absorbed by the body, it is recommended that they be cooked in order to get the full benefit. Heat changes the chemistry of carrots, making the nutrients available to the body.

Bran is a good source of fiber. But do not eat it raw. It may scratch the wall of the stomach or intestine. Bran becomes soft with cooking, and then can be eaten safely. (Bamboo shoots and carrots are naturally soft and act gently to stretch the intestines.)

FOOD COMBINATIONS

DO combine your food wisely, taking into consideration the Five Tastes, the Energy Levels, and the Acid-Alkaline balance of the food you eat. See Tables II, III, IV, V, VI, VII, IX, and X.

It will come as a surprise to many people that some foods become mildly toxic in our bodies when eaten in certain combinations. These toxic combinations are beef eaten with onion; banana with sweet potato, which produces dizziness; and crab with persimmon, which poisons the intestines.

FRUITS

DO eat fruits raw when they are fruits with thick skins. First, however, the fruit should be peeled—even apples—because worms live under the skin. In addition, the skin of anything is hard to digest.

The seeds of the fruit should also be eaten. The body can benefit greatly from the contents of the seeds as well as the "heart"—the center of the fruit nearest the seeds, such as an apple core. The heart and seeds contain laetrile (as well as countless other as-yet-unidentified things) which cleans the liver and detoxifies the body.

In ancient China, a person exposed to too much smoke was given apples to eat as a way of detoxifying the liver. (The liver is the body's filter for all solid substances.) These days apples can be used in the same way when a person is exposed to air pollution or smoke inhalation.

Any type of smoke is poisonous to the body, including tobacco and marijuana smoke. Marijuana is especially toxic because of the way it is smoked: the smoke is drawn into the lungs and held there until it is completely absorbed into the bloodstream. After five minutes of marijuana smoking, the liver is overloaded with toxins and unable to handle them anymore. If a person is a heavy user of marijuana, within one month 10% of the liver will be permanently damaged. Smoking marijuana is, therefore, definitely not recommended.

ILLNESS

DO eat foods that supply readily available forms of energy. This way energy is conserved for fighting disease-causing agents and for healing, instead of being of concentrated on digestion. One food that is extremely easy to digest is Rice Soup (see recipe). It can be combined with bits of fish, chicken soup, vegetables, anything that is not taxing for the digestive system to process.

LIQUID INTAKE

Again, and I continue to repeat this because it is the single most important point in this book, DO LIMIT YOUR INTAKE OF LIQUIDS. Healthy human kidneys can comfortably filter six cups of liquid a day. Any more is stored in the body tissues, causing water retention. If water retention is allowed to persist, this water in the body becomes jelly-like and collects the wastes and germs in the body, poisoning the tissues of the body in turn. The nerves are particularly affected. Not only are they squeezed under the pressure of the water retained under the skin, but they are also attacked by the germs and poisons existing in that stagnant water. This is why people who suffer chronic water retention also feel nervous and edgy.

MARGARINE

DO NOT eat margarine. As I said before, it is even worse than butter for your system. As a result of the process by which it is produced, margarine remains the same under any condition. It even remains unaltered in freezing conditions.

MEAT

DO eat meat, if your body needs the high energy level that only animal protein can supply.

However, there are problems connected with eating animal protein these days because of the stimulants and growth hormones which are so widely used by the growers and producers of the meats we buy in our stores. Also, individual animals carry various diseases, especially tuberculosis in beef, in their bloodstreams. These unnatural additives and disease organisms can have detrimental effects on our own health if we consume them.

Therefore it is a must that the meat we eat be treated and prepared in such a way so as to cleanse it of its harmful components, leaving only the beneficial tissues for our consumption. Treating the meat correctly does not lessen its nutritive value. The protein and tissues remain intact; only the harmful parts are disposed of.

Here is the correct method for preparing meat for cooking:

1. Place the meat in a shallow dish and cover it with water.

2. Soak the meat for several hours, changing the water frequently as the blood is soaked out of the tissues. (The harmful toxins and germs are only in the blood, not the tissues themselves.)

3. When all the blood is soaked out of the meat (when the soaking water no longer turns pink) drain the water off the meat.

4. Slice the meat very thinly.

5. Return the meat to the shallow dish for a second soaking period. This time cover the slices of meat with any strong alcoholic beverage such as whisky, gin, vodka, or brandy. (This will remove any remaining germs or parasites in the meat. Many of these organisms resist heat well and will not succumb to ordinary cooking.) A little soy sauce and "Five Spices" (a blend of spices available at specialty stores and Chinese markets) may be added to the marinade. This marinade will give lots of flavor to the meat as well as treat it.

6. Marinate the meat for about 30 minutes.

7. Cook the meat quickly at high temperatures, without burning it, until is is completely well-done (no pink flesh left).

If you have any qualms about killing any organism for food, please read the Preface.

DO not eat animal fat. Any type of animal fat, including dairy products such as butter and cheese, contains high levels of cholesterol. This cholesterol clogs the honeycomb structures in the liver, interfering with or blocking the organ's function, which can then lead to serious liver diseases. The reason is that the animal has already converted its food into fat, and this fat will not melt once it is inside the body. Instead it collects in the liver. In addition, cholesterol collects in the blood vessels where it can create dangerous problems for the heart.

Beef fat is the worst kind of fat. It will only melt or break down when heated to temperatures over 600°—this explains why it is used in heavy industries to grease machines.

Beef must be sliced thin, cooked well-done over high heat, and its fat be allowed to drain off as it cooks. Of course, when choosing meat, pick the leanest possible and trim off all fat before cooking.

Pork fat is more suitable for human consumption, because it breaks down or melts very easily inside the body. Unfortunately, pork is very toxic since pigs do not perspire and cannot rid their bodies of toxins. So the toxins collect in the body tissues of the pig.

We do need fat in our diet. Its purpose is to clean and lubricate the liver, kidneys, and lungs—the three filters of the body—but it must not clog them, as we have mentioned before. The best fat for this purpose is cold-pressed sesame oil. It is the lightest of all vegetable oils; it is even water-soluble. Some people object to the heavy, pervasive tastes and odors of vegetable oils. These can be eliminated by browning a few slices of fresh ginger root in the oil before cooking. This will purify the oil, and also rid the oil of most of the odor and flavor.

NATURAL FOODS

DO eat food in its natural state. Chemically processed foods cannot be metabolized properly by the body, and the toxins from the food remain in the system. Our bodies know how to use only whole, natural foods. Chemical additives and preservatives are not God-given; they are man-made. Avoid MSG, commercially processed sugar (raw, untreated sugar is a good food and contains many necessary nutrients), and decaffeinated coffee (the chemicals used in the decaffeinating process make it even worse than plain coffee!)

SHELLFISH

DO NOT eat shellfish in warm weather. Some foods are toxic even when eaten alone, and shellfish is very toxic when eaten in warm weather. (For some people, a particular shellfish can be toxic to their systems *any* time of the year.) This is because shellfish, such as clams and oysters, like cold water. When the water warms up in summer, these animals are sick and suffering, and their bodies are congested. To protect themselves, their bodies have to fight back, and to do this they produce a hormone which helps them relieve the effects of the heat.

While this hormone is good for the shellfish, it is harmful to our bodies. This hormone aggravates the hidden trouble spots in our bodies, such as acne, neuritis, and infections. For this reason, it makes good sense to avoid these foods in the summer and whenever you are already sick.

SKIN MUSHROOM

Another ingredient used in Chinese cooking deserves special mention. It is a fungus, known as the skin mushroom or "cloud ears" which grows on pine trees. Being bitter, according to the Five Element Theory, the benefit of its nutrients goes to the heart. And it too cleans up the wastes and cholesterol that collect in the bloodstream. If included in the daily diet, as it is in China, it can prevent heart disease—which is virtually non-existent in China.

An equally important role the skin mushroom plays is that of a cleansing agent for the small intestine. There are tiny pores in the walls of the small intestine where nutrients are absorbed. Over time, these pores or minute holes can become blocked by various things such as the tiny poultry hairs. (Hair is never digested. When preparing poultry, wash it well and inspect it carefully for any hairs. A pair of tweezers works well in removing these hairs.)

When it is digested, part of the skin mushroom is absorbed (it goes to clean the bloodstream, as mentioned before) and the rest passes through the small intestine in a sticky, gelatinous state, molding itself into the folds and curves of the intestine. As it passes through the small intestine, it picks up the little hairs and germs, and carries them out in the stools, thereby unblocking the pores. The skin mushroom is the only food that has this ability, so it is a very important part of our diet.

TOFU

DO include tofu (soybean curd) in your daily diet. Tofu is an excellent source of lecithin, which has the ability to clean out the cholesterol that has collected in our blood vessels. It is also an excellent source of protein and fiber. Under normal circumstances, tofu sits for days in water where germs may have a chance to establish themselves. For this reason, always cook tofu before eating it. If tofu tastes sour, it is spoiled. Do not eat it. Tofu has a very bland taste and texture, and combines well with a variety of dishes.

TOXIC FOODS

There has been much consternation over this topic. Almost every-day there are reports of precious resources being poisoned by man. PCB, mercury, aluminum, lead, copper, radiation, pesticides, to mention a few, are found in oceans, reservoirs, soil, etc., and consequently in vegetables, fish, livestock, and other food sources. Our territory of safe food consumption seems to shrink all the time, and more and more people seem to get sick from allergies to poi-soned foods. As if to add fuel to the fire, the situation grows more serious day after day. This may seem true at first thought, and man may be responsible for many ills, but further probing into the workings of nature will reveal that toxins exist naturally. The earth is composed of 93 naturally occurring, mostly toxic, elements. Almost every organism on earth—all composites of these earthly elements—is capable of combining elements to produce substances that are poisonous to other organisms, e.g., certain kinds of chrysan-themum flowers are capable of synthesizing pesticides, certain snakes are capable of secreting poison in their fangs. Snakebites are very toxic to human beings, but human bites are toxic to snakes as well. Everything works together in the universe only to benefit those who know how. It is God's will. But since the human race has been able to adapt to and tolerate toxins for so long, it can continue to tolerate toxins, present conditions notwithstanding.

One evening a few years ago, three doctors expressing three different points of view (conventional, holistic, and Taoistic) were invited to speak at the University of Oregon at Eugene about survival. The first speaker was the head of the health sciences department, and the main points of his speech were that the human body could not distinguish natural foods and drugs from synthetic foods and drugs (both kinds were accepted by the body) and that human beings could eat anything. He cited many nonagenarians who lived on nothing but the so-called junk foods. The second speaker, a famous man who spoke from a holistic standpoint, said that we were in the midst of a junk food crisis, because people were dying from eating junk food. As a reflection of the criticalness of the situation, he gave the following example: after his wife returned from the supermarket with bag loads of grocery, he went through the grocery and threw everything away, because nothing was safe to eat. Both doctors held completely contradictory views, and both supplied scientific evidence in support of their views. I was the third speaker. After saying both doctors were right, I said that since we were already living in a toxic environment with no hope of immediate change, we should learn to adapt to it, and that the key to our adaptation lay in our livers, which, when strengthened, could help us tolerate even great amounts of toxins.

We can not avoid toxins for as long as we live. Therefore, we must thank God for giving us a liver, for our livers are toxin filters and "detoxifiers", without which we can not survive. If our livers are strong and work well, we can tolerate everything; if not, we will sicken and die. To the present toxin problems, there are two solutions: 1) Food balance and 2) Strong livers. If meals are balanced, toxins from different foods balance one another, thus minimizing the toxicity of the entire meal, and giving us another cause for learning how to combine foods wisely and properly. To strengthen the liver's function, in my opinion, junk food should be eaten once in a while to temper its functions. Because living strictly on pure foods in pure environments can weaken the liver's ability to tolerate toxins, a single exposure to toxins can be fatal. To keep tolerance levels at a maximum we must exercise, or train, the liver by giving it chances to eliminate toxins, or in other words, by eating some junk food. Of course in Taoism, herbal combinations play a great role in strengthening the liver and neutralizing toxins and radiation. A final important tip is to avoid saturated fats, which can clog the liver. Given these methods of dealing with toxins, I hope everyone will rest more assured about toxins, and not panic, limit food intake, or become too weak, so that there will be no basis for the joke about finding healthier looking people in front of the junk food place instead of in front of the health food place.

VEGETABLES

DO cook all vegetables at least briefly. Cooked food is easier for the body to digest and assimilate because the chemical change that takes place during cooking assists the body in its digestive processes. Raw food tends to overstimulate the small intestine. Moreover, there are many harmful organisms residing in the vegetables and fruits we eat, as well as in meat.

By simply parboiling most vegetables very briefly (less than one minute) in boiling water, most of the organisms are killed. This way very little nutrition is lost and the color of the vegetable or fruit remains attractive.

Some strong vegetables (green beans, for example) need to be chopped and stir-fried for a few minutes in a small amount of oil. This will draw out the water in the vegetable, thereby killing the organisms in that water. This method is also more tasty than the parboiling method.

Some weak vegetables, such as lettuce, can be eaten raw by most people. Since everyone has a different tolerance for different foods, some people can experience discomfort when eating such vegetables. If you experience heartburn after eating a salad, this is a signal that raw vegetables are not for you. Even these weak vegetables contain unfriendly organisms. By soaking the vegetable in vinegar and water for a few minutes, then rinsing with cold water, these unwelcome guests will be removed.

WATER OR LIQUID WITH MEALS

DO not drink liquids with your meals. To drink too much liquid of any kind with food is tantamount to washing the food down. This prevents the mixing of saliva with the food during the chewing process. Saliva is a natural regulator of the acidity (pH) of the stomach. Without its being mixed into each bite of food, the acidity or pH of the stomach can be upset, thus interfering with digestion. Often gas or belching during or after a meal is a result of too much liquid taken with the food and improper pH of the stomach.

DO drink a small glass of wine with your dinner if you wish as this aids in the digestion of the food.

WHITE AND BROWN RICE

DO eat white rice and in general grains which have been milled to remove the shell around the seed. The shell of brown rice is very hard to cook, chew, and digest. Although brown rice is a good source of nutrients, none of its nutrients will be missed if white rice is eaten with dishes balanced in the Five Tastes as previously discussed. You may find that white rice complements your meal better, since white rice plays an important role as an equalizer.

Rice equalizes, complements, and neutralizes any dish, so that upset stomachs, heartburn, or ulcers are prevented. It is especially good for those who have too much stomach acid. So eating rice with your meals will make any meal safe. Bread, on the other hand, encourages the stomach to make acid. And if bread is made with bleached flour, it can be poisonous.

WHOLE FOODS

DO eat whole food. Follow God's wisdom and eat the *original* food. Believing that vitamin tablets can make up for the vital food missed in a reducing diet is a mistake. Our bodies have the knowledge they need to deal with food in its original form. Highly concentrated vitamin pills are foreign to the make-up and inner workings of the body, and pass through, largely unassimilated, into the urine.

PART IV

7

Recipes for Weight Control and Full Nutrition

Every one of the recipes in this section exactly follows the Taoist principles and theories of nutrition and balance, including the Five Elements and Five Tastes, energy (hot/cold) balance, pH balance, and the proper preparation and combination of foods. As you eat and enjoy these meals, you will have the full assurance and satisfaction that you are eating food which will help you lose weight as it provides full, balanced nutrition. You will literally be eating your way to health, energy, and a more vigorous and enjoyable life. Good Eating!!

THE FOUR PRINCIPLES OF A HEALTHFUL MEAL

There are four basic principles for recipes:

1. Good flavor
2. Good aroma
3. Good appearance
4. Good nutrition

Every dish must meet these four principles. If any recipe is lacking in any of these requirements, it is not a good recipe.

There is a universal principle for eating. Let us refer to Genesis—after man was created. The first order of God to man is the principle of eating: "Of every tree in the garden thou mayest freely eat." But in consideration of one tree, called the "tree of knowledge", God said "Thou shalt not eat of it, for in the day that thou eatest thereof thou shalt surely die."

God's command may be interpreted as an order to eat every tree, not to stick to one. If man eats only one type of food, he will die, because man needs everything to support his body, and one food cannot cover the needs of man. The human body is the microcosm and the universe is the macrocosm. Of course, after the flood, God added animals to man's nutrition list.

Eve chose to use her own concept of the universal principle, which is against the true principle. When she saw that the tree of knowledge was good for food, "that it is was pleasant to the eyes, and a tree to be desired to make one wise, she took of the fruit thereof, and did eat, and gave also unto her husband with her, and he did eat". The human concept—Eve's concept—is that one tree covers everything. The universal principle is eating everything but one thing. these recipes follow the universal principle. I shall enlarge upon the food territory as much as possible, so we may use the true wisdom to eat them properly in order to prolong life. I hope the readers are always aware of this principle, for there are many diet plans on the market that go against the true principle. Therefore the diets are not beneficial for longevity or balance of health.

GENERAL COMMENTS

All broths can be used in all recipes. For instance, they can be used as sauces, soups, etc. The flavor and nutritive value of any recipe is improved thus. One special use: freeze the broth, cut the jelly-like broth into cubes and use them in salads.

Always when cooking chicken broth, you are better off buying chicken that has been raised without chemical stimulants. When cooking chicken, the fat under the skin (yellow and rubbery) must be scraped away, because the fat is very abundant.

Bones can be obtained from butchers. Usually they are just thrown away. When you ask for bones you can get many of them for a very cheap price. Bones must be cooked until they are very, very soft in order to retrieve their hidden nutrients.

Cheese. Please use cheese made with skim milk.

Fish. Catfish contains the most nutrition, but all fish provide good amounts. If you prefer shellfish to other fish, by all means use shellfish. Be sure to remove all sand from clams, mussels, and other shellfish. For shrimp make an incision along the entire center back of the shrimp. Remove the dark artery of the shrimp which contains waste products. Note: Use no shellfish with surface blemishes.

Vegetables. Seaweeds are very important for the thyroid gland. Mushrooms are equally important as a cleansing food.

Always rinse rice well. Since each rice kernel is sometimes coated with talcum for cosmetic or packaging reasons, and talcum can cause cancer, it is wise to rinse rice several times before cooking. This can be done by placing the desired amount of rice in a large pot, adding twice the amount of water to cover the rice, and swirling the rice with your hand. When the water turns cloudy, let the rice settle and pour off the water (it does not matter if a little water must remain to prevent pouring rice down the drain). Repeat these steps again until the water is quite clear. It is best to avoid instant rice.

Soak and prepare all meat according to instructions on page 113.

Use raw sugar wherever possible when sugar is called for. Raw sugar is in a natural state and is therefore free of chemicals, making it easier for the body to assimilate.

Always eat three meals a day. Keep in mind to eat like a *king* for breakfast, a *queen* for lunch, and a *prince* for dinner.

SAMPLE DAILY DIET PLAN
FOR 100 DAY DIET

You can choose your breakfast, lunch, and dinner by following the following recipes. All dishes can be combined with rice, a small amount of bread or rolls, etc. Be sure to eat, everyday, 1 apple and 2 oranges or ½-1 grapefruit and 1 banana, or other seasonal fruits (8 oz.) like cherries, melons, etc. For example:

Breakfast: Mushroom and Egg
           Toast
           1 cup nonfat milk
           1 banana
Lunch: Sandwich with Barbecued Beef Tongue
           1 orange
           1 cup tea
Dinner: 1 cup/bowl fish soup
           Cucumber salad
           Wine Vinegar Chicken
           1 bowl rice

This is just one day's suggestion. I have listed recipes that, with imagination, can make up a 100-day diet plan.

Eating is the most important part of life for healing and maintenance. It is also the most important and best way to enjoy life. One must spend as much time as possible for eating. After your meal has been prepared, sit down, relax, and slowly enjoy your meal.

I repeat.

> *Eat on time.*
> *Eat well.*
> *Eat slowly.*
> *Eat balanced meals.*

And enjoy. Eating is the biggest blessing from God.

BROTH BASE FOR ALL DISHES

There are three soup bases:

Chicken broth
Bone broth
Fish broth

Chicken Broth

1 chicken, whole

1 green onion

2 Tbs. cooking wine

2 slices ginger

1 Tbs. salt, or to taste

10 cups water

Chop whole chicken into about 2″ squares. Mix it in a bowl with the onion, ginger, salt, and wine. Let it sit 20-30 minutes.

Put 10 cups of water in a pot and bring it to a boil. Add the chicken and other ingredients to the water, bring to boil.

Reduce heat and simmer for 2 hours until the bones are soft.

Remove from heat and cool for 1 hour. Then strain the broth through a strainer, removing all large, solid particles.

Refrigerate overnight. Next morning remove the layer of hardened fat which has collected on top of the broth. (This layer is more opaque than the broth layer underneath.) The broth is of a jelly-like consistency. It can be reheated and added to all recipes to improve taste.

Bone Broth

  3 lbs. pork or chicken bones

  1 Tbs. salt

  2 slices ginger

  1 green onion

  4 Tbs. wine

Follow Chicken Broth instructions. Simmer till bones are soft. Then mash the bones and strain.

Fish Broth

  2 lbs. catfish (whole, scaled, and gutted)

  ¼ tsp. pepper

  3 slices ginger

  1 green onion

  4 Tbs. cooking wine

To cook, follow Chicken Broth instructions.

SOUPS

All recipes serve 4 people.

Seaweed Soup

   2 oz. pork, thinly sliced

   1 Tbs. green onion, chopped

   1 slice ginger

   ½ tsp. wine

   ½ tsp. cornstarch

   ½ cup chicken broth

   3 cups water

   1 tsp. salt, or to taste

   2 sheets seaweed, dried

Combine pork, onion, ginger, wine, and cornstarch in a bowl. Mix well.

Let sit 15 minutes.

Combine broth and water and bring to boil in pot. While boiling, add salt and pork mixture.

Tear seaweed and add to pot.

Boil for a few minutes. Serve.

Benefits
This soup is a tonic for the thyroid. It is good for the metabolism, cleanses the blood, and purifies and adjusts hormones.

131

Fish Soup

4-5 oz. fish fillet, sliced

1 tsp. cornstarch

½ tsp. salt, or to taste

½ tsp. green onion, minced

1 Tbs. wine

½ cup fish broth

3 cups water

¼ cup bamboo shoots or cucumbers, sliced

½ tsp. salt, or to taste

2 Tbs. cornstarch

1 Tbs. water

½ Tbs. sesame oil, hot pressed

pepper to taste

Combine fish, 1 tsp. cornstarch, salt, onion, and wine in bowl and mix well, let sit.

Combine broth and 3 cups water, bring to boil, then add above mixture, bamboo, and salt.

Mix 2 Tbs. cornstarch with 1 Tbs. water in a small dish, then add to soup, stirring slightly.

Sprinkle on sesame oil and pepper and serve.

Benefits
This soup is rich in protein and vitamins. It also rejuvenates, and fights cancer. It builds the body as well as beautifies.

Hot and Sour Soup

6 pieces skin mushrooms (black fungus) from Oriental
food store

10 pieces Lily flowers, dried, from Oriental food store

½ cup chicken broth

3 cups water

⅔ package tofu, rinsed and cubed

1 green onion, finely chopped

10 thin slices of lean pork

½ tsp. pepper, or to taste

¼ cup bamboo shoots, sliced

1 oz. shrimp, dried, from Oriental food store

1 tsp. salt, or to taste

½ tsp. sesame oil, hot pressed

1-3 Tbs. vinegar, or to taste

1 egg, beaten

1½ Tbs. cornstarch

1 Tbs. water

Soak mushrooms and Lily flowers in water until they are soft.
Remove hard parts of mushrooms and slice. Cut Lily flowers into
half length.

Combine chicken broth and 3 cups water in a pot. Bring to boil. Add
all other ingredients except egg, vinegar, and cornstarch. Cook on
low heat for 10-15 minutes. Check taste. Then add vinegar.

Stir soup in clockwise direction. While stirring, slowly and sparingly pour in egg. The egg will form ribbons. Finally, mix cornstarch with 1 Tbs. water. Add to the soup. Keep stirring until soup thickens.

Serve hot.

Benefits
This soup is excellent for common colds, coughing, poor circulation, bronchitis, arthritis, sluggish liver, indigestion, hormone imbalance, and toxic blood. It also fights cholesterol.

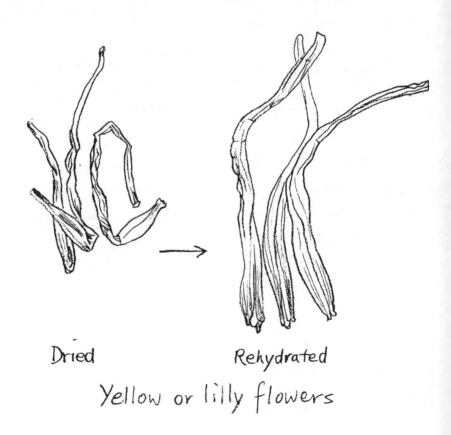

Dried   Rehydrated

Yellow or lilly flowers

Corn and Chicken Soup

   1 egg, beaten

   2 chicken breasts, ground

   4 oz. can cream of corn, unsweetened

   3 cups water

   ½ cup bone broth

   1 tsp. salt, or to taste

   1½ Tbs. cornstarch

   1 Tbs. water

   2 Tbs. milk, lowfat or nonfat

Mix egg and chicken well in bowl. Set aside.

Combine 3 cups water and broth in pot. Add corn and salt and stir.

Bring to boil.

Mix cornstarch and 1 Tbs. water well in a small bowl.

Add cornstarch mixture to pot and stir. While stirring in clockwise direction, add chicken mixture. Bring to boil again.

Remove from heat. Serve.

Benefits
This soup is rich in vitamin E. It increases sexual energy. It also strengthens the heart and is rich in all other nutrients.

Tofu and Spinach Soup

   3 cups water

   ½ cup vegetable broth

   1 package tofu, rinsed and cubed

   ½ bunch spinach, cleaned and chopped

   1 tomato, peeled, sliced, and seeds removed

   1 tsp. salt, or to taste

   ¼ tsp. sesame oil, hot pressed

   pepper to taste

Combine water and broth in a pot. Bring to boil.

Add to pot tofu, spinach, tomato, and salt.

Add sesame oil and sprinkle on pepper. Serve.

Benefits
This soup is food for the brain. It nourishes the brain as well as soothes the heart, and fights cholesterol as well as cleans the blood vessels. The soup is rich in protein and other nutrients.

SALAD DRESSINGS

Spicy Oil with Lemon

¼ cup sesame oil, cold pressed

¼ cup fresh lemon juice

½-¾ tsp. salt (to taste)

¼ tsp. ground black pepper

Combine oil, lemon juice, salt, and pepper. Shake vigorously.

Refrigerate. Shake well before serving.

Oil and Vinegar with Soy

6 Tbs. sesame oil

1½ Tbs. soy sauce

3 Tbs. white wine vinegar

1 tsp. white pepper

1 tsp. garlic, minced

½-¾ tsp. salt (to taste)

Combine all ingredients well. Refrigerate. Shake before serving.

Spicy Vinegar and Oil

   1 tsp. Dijon style mustard

   ¼ cup sesame oil, cold pressed

   ¼ cup white wine vinegar

   ¾ tsp. dill

   ¾ tsp. thyme

   ½ tsp. raw sugar

   1 tsp. garlic, minced

   ¾ tsp. chives

   ½-¾ tsp. salt (to taste)

Combine all ingredients. Shake vigorously.

Refrigerate. Shake well before serving.

Cucumber/Lemon Yogurt

¼ cup plain yogurt

2 Tbs. sesame oil

2 Tbs. fresh lemon juice

2 Tbs. cucumber, pureed

2 Tbs. onion, minced

1 tsp. fresh mint, minced

1 tsp. fresh parsley, minced

½-¾ tsp. salt (to taste)

½ tsp. black pepper, ground

Combine all ingredients. Shake vigorously. Let sit 6 hours.

Refrigerate. Dressing can last 1 week.

Blue Cheese

¼ cup sesame oil, cold pressed

2 tsp. white wine vinegar

2 oz. blue cheese

6 Tbs. heavy cream

1 tsp. Worcestershire sauce

1 tsp. onion, minced

¼ tsp. black pepper, ground

½-¾ tsp. salt (to taste)

Combine all ingredients. Mix well. Refrigerate.

Egg and Oil

1 egg yolk

½ tsp. mustard powder

½-¾ tsp. salt (to taste)

2 tsp. fresh lemon juice

¾ cup sesame oil, cold pressed

1 tsp. white pepper

1 tsp. cinnamon (optional)

Beat egg yolk for 2 minutes. Blend in mustard powder, salt, and lemon juice. Continue mixing for 1 minute. While mixing, add sesame oil, a little at a time. Add white pepper and cinnamon (optional).

Sour Cream with Spices

¼ cup sour cream

2 Tbs. Egg and Oil dressing (without cinnamon)

1 Tbs. tarragon white wine vinegar

2 tsp. fresh lemon juice

1 tsp. garlic, minced

1 Tbs. parsley, minced

1 tsp. chives

2 tsp. green onion, finely chopped

2 tsp. anchovy paste

½-¾ tsp. salt (to taste)

1 tsp. white pepper

Combine all ingredients. Blend well. Refrigerate.

BREAKFAST DISHES

All recipes serve 4 people.

Many of these recipes can be prepared the night before, to simplify cooking the following morning. All breakfast recipes given here are intended to satisfy full nutritional needs, and are excellent energizers. Sometimes a bit of tea can be made to accompany your morning meal. Green onion does not affect the breath.

Fried Rice with Eggs

    4 Tbs. vegetable oil

    4 eggs, beaten

    4 cups cooked rice

    1 green onion, minced

    1 Tbs. cooked, crumbled bacon or chopped ham

    ½ tsp. salt

In pan, heat vegetable oil and scramble eggs. Add rice. Then add salt and bacon. Taste. Add more salt if needed. Add green onion.

Stir fry for 3-4 minutes. Serve.

Special Benefit
This breakfast is highly recommended for those who do heavy physical work and need solid food to fill up the stomach in the morning.

Fish with Egg

4 oz. fish

½ tsp. salt

1 Tbs. cornstarch

1 Tbs. wine

1 tsp. soy sauce

⅛ tsp. black pepper

1 green onion, chopped

½ tsp. salt

½ cup fish broth

½ tsp. sesame oil, hot pressed

4 eggs

Combine fish, ½ tsp. salt, cornstarch, wine, soy sauce, pepper, and fish broth in bowl and set aside.

Beat eggs and add other ½ tsp. salt.

Combine eggs with fish mixture. Add green onion.

Put in double boiler, steam 15 minutes and serve.

Mushrooms and Eggs

    12 fresh mushrooms, medium sized

    12 skin mushrooms (black mushrooms), soaked and drained

    4 Tbs. vegetable oil

    1 Tbs. green onion, chopped

    1 slice ginger, finely chopped

    ¾ tsp. garlic, minced

    1 Tbs. soy sauce

    1 tsp. sugar

    1 tsp. vinegar

    4 eggs, well beaten

Slice all mushrooms and stir them with 1 Tbs. of vegetable oil. Set aside in bowl.

In pan, heat rest of vegetable oil, add onion, ginger, and garlic. Then add mushrooms, soy sauce, sugar, and vinegar and stir fry.

At last minute, add eggs, stir, and serve.

Bamboo, Beef, and Eggs

8 oz. lean beef, sliced

1 Tbs. wine

1 Tbs. cornstarch

2 Tbs. soy sauce

¼ tsp. salt

1 tsp. sugar

1 green onion, cut into 1″ lengths

4 eggs

2 slices ginger, very finely chopped

4 Tbs. vegetable oil

1 small can bamboo shoots, sliced

Combine beef, wine, cornstarch, soy sauce, salt, and sugar. Mix in ginger and bamboo shoots.

In pan, heat 2 Tbs. vegetable oil, add beef mixture, and stir fry until beef is well done.

In pan, heat 2 Tbs. vegetable oil, stir fry onion, add eggs, and scramble until done.

Combine eggs with beef and serve. Or stir fry onions, add to beef mixture, and scramble eggs with beef mixture.

Chicken Breakfast

2 chicken breasts, sliced into 4 pieces

4 Tbs. soy sauce

2 Tbs. wine

½ Tbs. sugar

1 Tbs. cornstarch

1 Tbs. sesame oil, hot pressed

4 eggs

8 Tbs. vegetable oil

1 green onion, cut into 1″ lengths

2 slices ginger, chopped

Combine chicken, soy sauce, wine, sugar, cornstarch, and sesame oil.

Mix well in bowl and set aside for 20 minutes. Then separate chicken from juice, saving the juice.

In pan, heat 4 Tbs. of vegetable oil, sautee onion and ginger, and fry chicken until done.

In another pan, heat 4 Tbs. of vegetable oil, drop in 1 egg and fry.

Transfer 1 piece of chicken to top of fried egg. Do the same with the other three eggs and pieces of chicken.

Heat juice you have earlier separated from chicken. Pour juice over chicken and serve.

Toast with Cheese

8 slices bread

8 oz. cheddar cheese, shredded

4 Tbs. vegetable oil

4 eggs, beaten

2 cups skim or low fat milk

1 Tbs. green onion, chopped

½ tsp. salt

4 oz. shrimp or ground lean meat

Cube bread. Spread vegetable oil evenly in a 13" × 9" baking tray. Place bread in tray and sprinkle on shredded cheese.

Combine beaten eggs, milk, green onion, and salt and pour over bread.

Spread shrimp or meat over top of mixture.

Bake at 350° for 45-60 minutes. Check for doneness and serve.

Dish can be wrapped in aluminum foil for overnight refrigeration and reheated the next morning.

Spinach and Egg Puff

½ lb. spinach, cleaned and chopped

4 eggs, beaten

¼ tsp. salt

1 cup chicken broth

1 tsp. vegetable oil

Combine eggs, salt, and chicken broth and mix well.

Grease a large bowl with vegetable oil.

Combine spinach with egg mixture and pour into bowl.

Place in top section of double boiler and steam 18 minutes and serve.

Meat and Egg Pie

½ lb. lean beef

1 tsp. salt

¼ tsp. ginger, powdered

1 Tbs. wine

1 Tbs. cornstarch

4 eggs

1 green onion, chopped

1 tsp. sesame oil, hot pressed

Combine beef, salt, ginger, wine, and cornstarch in bowl. Mix well.

Drop eggs on beef mixture.

Place mixture in top section of double boiler and steam for 30 minutes.

Check for doneness. Garnish with green onion and sesame oil. Serve.

Egg Roll with Fish

½ lb. filet rock cod, ground

¼ tsp. black pepper

1 tsp. wine

1 Tbs. cornstarch

4 eggs, each beaten separately

4 Tbs. vegetable oil

1 carrot, quartered lengthwise

1 tsp. salt

Combine cod, pepper, wine, cornstarch, and salt in bowl. Mix well and let sit.

In pan, heat 1 Tbs. vegetable oil, stir fry cod mixture 5 minutes, drain and set aside.

In another pan, heat 1 tsp. of oil, add 1 beaten egg and spread over bottom of pan, and cook to form a crepe-like omelette.

Fill with ¼ of cod mixture and roll up. Insert a carrot stick in the middle of the roll. Repeat process with remaining eggs and fish mixture.

Refrigerate rolls overnight.

Next day heat by baking at 325° for 15 minutes.

Serves 4.

LUNCH DISHES

Lunches should be accompanied by fresh vegetables and fruits. All recipes serve 4 people.

Barbecued Tongue (see dinner recipe).

Barbecued Beef Shank (see dinner recipe).

Barbecued Cha Shao

    4 lb. pork

    ½ cup soy sauce

    ¼ cup ketchup

    ¼ tsp. ground cinnamon

    1 Tbs. salt

    1 Tbs. sugar

    1 whole garlic, minced

    1 stick ginger

    1 green onion, quartered

    2 Tbs. wine

    3 Tbs. vegetable oil

Cut pork to 2″ thick.

Combine soy sauce, ketchup, cinnamon, salt, sugar, garlic, ginger, onion, and wine. Add pork and soak for 3 hours, turning pork occasionally.

Cook for ½ hour, then separate meat from juices. Cool.

In pan, heat vegetable oil, and fry pork until golden brown. Cool and thinly slice. Combine with juice. Serve.

Benefits
This dish supplies energy and nutrients. It is also a decongestant and detoxifier.

Rice with Meat

2 cups rice, uncooked

½ lb. completely lean ground meat, lamb, etc., or dried shrimp

1 carrot, peeled and diced

1 onion, diced

6 Tbs. ketchup

2 Tbs. vegetable oil

1 tsp. salt

3½ cups water

Wash rice. In pan, heat oil, sautee carrot and onion, and add rice, meat, ketchup, salt, and water.

(If you are using shrimp instead of meat, soak shrimp in boiling water twice, drain, and let sit 10 minutes before cooking.)

Bring to boil, reduce to low heat, cover and cook for ½ hour, stirring occasionally.

Benefits
This dish is an overall energizer and detoxifier. It is also suitable for dinner.

Spaghetti

4 oz. shrimp

1 Tbs. hot pressed sesame oil

½ lb. spaghetti

2 Tbs. vegetable oil

4 oz. ground lean meat

½ tsp. salt, or to taste

1 Tbs. wine

4 oz. fresh mushrooms, chopped

2 oz. roasted, unsalted peanuts, chopped

1 small, dried red pepper, chopped in half

3 Tbs. peanut butter

1 Tbs. vinegar

½ tsp. sugar

1 green onion, chopped

1 cup water or chicken stock

1 Tbs. cornstarch mixed with 2 Tbs. cold water

Soak shrimp in water, drain, and chop. Cook spaghetti, mix with sesame oil, and toss well.

In pan, heat vegetable oil, add shrimp, ground meat, salt, wine, and mushrooms and stir fry for 1-2 minutes or until meat is brown. Add peanuts, red pepper, peanut butter, vinegar, sugar, and green onion. Add 1 cup of water or chicken stock and cornstarch. Stir well. Combine with spaghetti and serve.

Benefits
This dish is an overall energy supplier and detoxifier. It is also suitable for dinner.

Curry Pie

1 box pie crust mix (follow mixing instructions on box)

¼ cup water

10-12 oz. lean pork or beef

1 Tbs. wine

1 Tbs. cornstarch

1 tsp. salt

1 Tbs. green onion, chopped

2-3 Tbs. curry powder

4 Tbs. vegetable oil

2 onions, diced

2 egg yolks

1 Tbs. water

Combine meat with wine, starch, salt, and green onion. Let sit 10 minutes.

In pan, heat 2 Tbs. vegetable oil, and stir fry meat mixture. Add curry powder, stir fry 5 minutes. Drain on paper towel. In pan, heat 2 Tbs. vegetable oil, sautee diced onion, and drain. Combine onions with meat mixture.

Roll mixed pie crust into a long "bar". Quarter. Pull each section into a long strand. Cut each section into tenths. Using a rolling pin, roll sections into round "tortillas".

Wrap enough of filling in two tortillas to make "pie". Pinch to seal edges. Make twenty "pies" this way.

Mix egg yolk and 1 Tbs. water well. Grease baking pan.

Brush surface of pies with egg yolk mixture. Place on pan with edges not touching.

Bake 15 minutes at 400°, then 10-15 minutes at 375° till golden brown. Serve.

Benefits
This dish is a stimulant. It is nutritious and energizing.

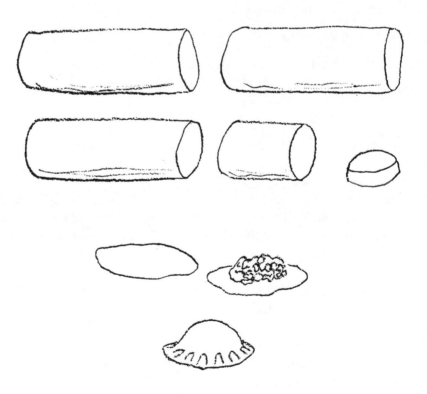

Living Salad

1 potato, cooked, skin removed, and mashed

1 hard boiled egg

1 tsp. hot pressed sesame oil

1 Tbs. sesame oil (cold pressed)

1 Tbs. mayonnaise

½ cup cooked macaroni

½ carrot, peeled, diced, and steamed for 3 minutes

1 apple, peeled and diced

½ cucumber, peeled and diced

½ tsp. salt

¼-½ tsp. pepper (to taste)

Separate the white and yolk of the egg. Dice the egg white.

Mash the yolk with sesame oil and mayonnaise.

Mix yolk mixture, diced egg white, potato, macaroni, carrot, apple, cucumber, salt and pepper. Serve.

Benefits
This salad provides many nutrients. It is both energizing and cleansing.

DINNER MEAT DISHES

All recipes serve 4 people.

Sesame oil used in recipes should be hot pressed for taste, except where noted. The amount of salt can be adjusted to one's taste in all recipes.

Barbecued Beef Shank

1 lb. beef shank

¼ cup soy sauce

2 cups water

2 tsp. salt

2 green onions, diced

2 slices ginger

1 stick cinnamon

¼ cup wine

hot pressed sesame oil

Clean beef and put in pot along with soy sauce, water, salt, onions, ginger, cinnamon, and wine. Bring to boil. Reduce to simmer, and simmer for 3 hours, stirring occasionally.

Cool and slice beef thinly. Sprinkle sesame oil over sliced meat and serve.

This dish may be eaten for lunch in a sandwich.

Benefits
This dish strengthens the nerves because it is rich in the appropriate nutrients. It supplies energy and contains hardly any fatty tissues.

Spicy Chicken

2 Tbs. sesame seeds

2 lb. chicken

3 Tbs. soy sauce

1 Tbs. wine

1 Tbs. vinegar

1 Tbs. green onion (chopped)

1 Tbs. garlic, finely diced

¼ tsp. chili powder (optional)

2 Tbs. hot pressed sesame oil (to taste)

1 tsp. salt

1 tsp. sugar

1 tsp. cornstarch

Roast sesame seeds.

Put enough water in pot to cover chicken, but do *not* add chicken. Bring to boil. Put chicken in pot. Bring to boil again. Reduce heat and simmer for 25 minutes or until done. Test for doneness by poking into flesh, making sure there is no blood. Cool. Remove skin and fat from chicken. Cut chicken into 2″ × 1″ pieces.

Combine seasonings (soy sauce, wine, vinegar, onion, garlic, chili powder, sesame oil, salt, sugar, and cornstarch) and add to chicken. Heat and serve. Sprinkle with sesame seeds.

Benefits
This dish is rich in nutrients. It strengthens and cleanses the lungs, and stimulates the large intestines and helps in elimination.

Sweet and Sour Pork Loin

1 lb. pork loin, sliced thinly

2 Tbs. cornstarch

1 Tbs. wine

¼ tsp. salt

1 green onion, chopped

2 slices ginger

2 cups vegetable oil

2½ Tbs. vinegar

1 tsp. salt

5½ Tbs. sugar

2 Tbs. tomato sauce

2 Tbs. cornstarch

½ cup water

1 tsp. soy sauce

½ cup green pepper, diced

½ cup carrot, diced

¼ cup pineapple, diced—or pineapple juice

Combine pork, 2 Tbs. cornstarch, wine, salt, onion, and ginger. Let sit in bowl 30 minutes.

Put oil in pan on high heat. Fry 2 pieces of pork at a time for 2-3 minutes. Drain on paper towel.

Combine vinegar, salt, sugar, tomato sauce, 2 Tbs. cornstarch, water, soy sauce, green pepper, carrot, and pineapple in saucepan. Cook, while constantly stirring, until sauce thickens.

Pour sauce over pork. Serve.

Benefits
This dish soothes the liver and pancreas. It nourishes as well as cleanses these organs.

Steamed Salmon

    4 fresh salmon steaks

    1 green onion, chopped

    2 slices ginger

    2 Tbs. wine

    1 tsp. salt

    1 Tbs. cornstarch

    4 oz. ground pork

    ½ tsp. salt

    1 tsp. wine

    ½ tsp. cornstarch

    ½ cup bamboo shoots, diced

    3 tsp. hot pressed sesame oil (or to taste)

    2 tsp. pepper

    pine leaves (optional)

Combine salmon, onion, ginger, 2 Tbs. wine, 1 tsp. salt, and 1 Tbs. cornstarch in bowl, mix well, and set aside. Combine pork, ½ tsp. salt, 1 tsp. wine, and ½ tsp. cornstarch in bowl, mix well, and set aside. Let both bowls set for 30 minutes. Press down salmon mixture, cover with layer of ½ cup bamboo shoots. Put pork mixture on top of bamboo shoots, spread out evenly.

Place in top part of double boiler, the bottom of which may be lined with pine leaves. Bring to boil for 3 minutes. Reduce to low heat and let steam for 30 minutes.

Garnish with sesame oil and pepper. Serve.

Benefits
This dish is a decongestant, and it is anti-inflammatory. It soothes and cleans the digestive system. The steam enhances flavor because it locks in flavor. When pine leaves are added to the boiling water, the resultant steam promotes longevity, enhances flavor, and increases nutrition.

Coconut Chicken

6 Tbs. vegetable oil

2 lb. chicken breasts or drumsticks

½ cup flour

1 Tbs. curry powder

2 Tbs. vegetable oil

2 green onions, chopped

3 cloves garlic, minced

1 lb. potatoes

1 cup milk

1 cup chicken broth

1 tsp. salt

2 Tbs. coconut juice

Heat 6 Tbs. vegetable oil in pan.

Roll chicken in flour until covered. Fry until golden brown. Drain on paper towel.

Mix curry powder with 2 Tbs. oil. Combine onions and garlic and sautee in curry/oil.

Remove skins from potatoes and cube. Fry in oil (from chicken frying) until golden brown. Drain on paper towel. Pour remaining oil from pan and return chicken to pan along with potatoes, onions, and garlic.

Combine milk, broth, salt, and coconut juice, and pour over chicken. Cover and simmer for 35-45 minutes, serve.

Benefits
This dish is rich in protein. It is good for the spleen- pancreas and digestion. It is especially nourishing for the kidneys and sexual organs.

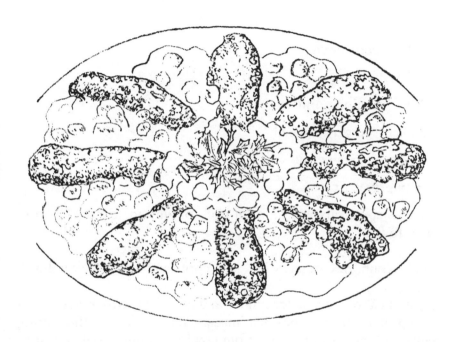

Sweet and Sour Shrimp

- 1 lb. shrimp
- 6 Tbs. ketchup
- 2 Tbs. raw sugar
- 1 Tbs. wine
- 1 tsp. salt
- 1 Tbs. cornstarch
- 1 Tbs. water
- 2 green onions, minced
- 2 slices ginger, minced
- 6 Tbs. vegetable oil
- ½ cup green peas

Remove epidermis and vein on back of shrimp. Rinse. Drain on paper towel.

Mix ketchup, raw sugar, wine, salt, cornstarch, and water in bowl.

In pan, heat oil and sautee onions and ginger for two minutes. Add shrimp and stir fry from 3 minutes. Pour oil out, letting shrimp remain in pan. Add mixture from bowl to shrimp, cook and stir 2 minutes. Put in serving dish.

Cook peas slightly, keeping green color. Add to shrimp mixture and serve.

Benefits
This dish is an overall energy food. People who have skin conditions should avoid it, however.

Tofu and Oyster Dish

4 oz. oysters or 4 oysters, washed thoroughly and chopped into small pieces

1 Tbs. cornstarch

1 tsp. wine

2 Tbs. vegetable oil

1 Tbs. garlic, minced

1 Tbs. green onion, minced

2 packages tofu, rinsed and cubed

2 Tbs. cornstarch

2 Tbs. water

¼ tsp. ginger, powdered

2 tsp. soy sauce

½ tsp. salt, or to taste

2 tsp. hot pressed sesame oil

Combine oysters, 1 Tbs. cornstarch and wine in bowl and set aside.

In pan, heat vegetable oil and sautee garlic and onion for 2 minutes. Add oysters and fry 3 minutes. Add tofu and gently stir fry for 5 minutes. Mix 2 Tbs. cornstarch with water in bowl, and add to oysters and tofu while still frying. Add ginger, soy sauce, and salt. Stir.

Remove from heat, garnish with sesame oil, and serve.

Benefits
This dish is a brain and sexual energy food. It helps dissolve tumors.

Family Style Tofu

½ lb. pork, thinly sliced

½ tsp. salt

1 Tbs. wine

1 Tbs. cornstarch

2 pieces dried black mushroom

3 Tbs. vegetable oil

1 package tofu, rinsed and sliced to 1½" × ½" × ½"

2 Tbs. vegetable oil

2 green onions, cut to 1" long strips

¼ cup bamboo shoots, diced

2 Tbs. soy sauce

1 tsp. brown sugar

Combine pork, salt, wine, and cornstarch in bowl. Set aside for 30 minutes.

Soak mushrooms in warm water thoroughly. Then slice.

In pan, heat 3 Tbs. oil and fry tofu until golden brown, then remove.

In 2 Tbs. oil sautee onions and bamboo shoots, being careful not to burn them. Then add mushrooms and pork mixture and stir fry for 5 minutes. Add tofu, soy sauce, and brown sugar, simmering until hot and blended. Serve.

Benefits
This dish helps the body fight cancer and cholesterol.

Wine Vinegar Chicken

1 cut-up chicken

1½ tsp. salt

1 Tbs. vegetable oil

1 Tbs. garlic, minced

⅓ cup wine vinegar

¼ cup wine

⅓ cup fresh lemon juice

4 Tbs. water

1 Tbs. ketchup

1 Tbs. cornstarch

1 Tbs. parsley, minced

¾ tsp. black pepper

Salt and pepper the chicken.

Place oil in pan, heat, and fry chicken until golden brown on all sides. Add garlic, wine vinegar, wine, lemon juice, water, and ketchup to chicken. Cover and cook over low heat for 15-20 minutes. Add cornstarch to thicken sauce.

Sprinkle parsley on top for garnish and serve.

Benefits
This dish soothes and cleans the gall bladder, liver, and nerves. It is good for the eyesight.

Roast in Peanut Butter Sauce

2 lb. English cut roast

½ tsp. salt

1 Tbs. wine

1 Tbs. cornstarch

1 green onion, chopped

1 slice ginger

1 tsp. garlic, powdered

½ lemon, juiced

3 oz. peanut butter

1 dried red pepper

1 Tbs. garlic, minced

1 onion, cubed

1 Tbs. soy sauce

2 Tbs. vegetable oil

Combine roast, salt, wine, cornstarch, green onion, ginger, and 1 tsp. garlic powder in bowl. Let sit 30 minutes.

In saucepan, heat vegetable oil, and sautee minced garlic, onion, and pepper.

Mix peanut butter well with a little water. Add to saucepan, bring to boil. Then add lemon juice.

Cut roast to ½″ thick slices. Pour sauce from saucepan on roast. Let sit 30 minutes.

Bake roast in oven at 325° for 30 minutes, or until well done.

Serve with juices. If there is not enough sauce, more can be made.

Benefits
This dish is a decongestant. It is also anti-inflammatory.

Beef Tripe

10-16 oz. tripe

1 Tbs. vegetable oil

1 onion, diced

1 stalk celery, chopped

½ tsp. salt, or to taste

¼ tsp. pepper

2 Tbs. cornstarch

1½ cups bone broth

1 Tbs. vinegar

1 green onion, diced

1 tsp. hot pressed sesame oil (or to taste)

Clean tripe. Place in a pot and add enough water to cover. Bring to a boil. Reduce to simmer. Cook 30 minutes.

Cool tripe, then slice.

In pan, sautee diced onion and celery in vegetable oil. Add salt, pepper, cornstarch, and broth. Then add vinegar.

Pour sauce on tripe. Garnish with green onion and sesame oil. Serve.

Benefits
This dish is good for the stomach, aiding in digestion. It strengthens the stomach tissue and duodenum.

Barbecued Tongue

2-3 lb. beef tongue

2 Tbs. vegetable oil

1 onion, cubed

½ cup ketchup

2 tsp. salt

1 Tbs. soy sauce

1 Tbs. vinegar

2 Tbs. wine

water

2 tsp. sesame oil

Clean beef tongue. Place in pot with enough water to cover. Bring to boil for 10 minutes. Skin should be white. Cool in a pan of cold water. Then, using knife, scrape off and discard white skin. Then drain off water.

In pan, heat vegetable oil and sautee onion. Add ketchup, salt, soy sauce, vinegar, and wine. Let cook 2 minutes. Add tongue. Then add water, cover, and cook for 3 hours over low heat. Check for doneness, then cool. Slice tongue to thin pieces.

Garnish with sesame oil and serve. Can be eaten for lunch in a sandwich.

Benefits
This dish is a heart food. It is good for strengthening the heart muscles and blood vessels.

DINNER VEGETABLE DISHES

All recipes serve 4 people.

String Bean Saute

  1 cup vegetable oil

  1 lb. string beans (ends removed, cleaned, and dried)

  3 Tbs. vegetable oil

  4 green onions, chopped

  2 slices ginger

  1 Tbs. garlic, minced

  4 Tbs. soy sauce

  1 Tbs. wine

  1 tsp. sugar

  salt to taste

In pan, heat 1 cup vegetable oil. Over medium heat fry beans till crinkly and brown. Drain on paper towel.

Slice long beans into thirds, short beans into halves.

In pan, heat 3 Tbs. vegetable oil and sautee onions, ginger, and garlic. Add beans, soy sauce, wine, sugar, and salt. Stir fry 1-2 minutes. Serve.

Benefits
This dish soothes the pancreas and helps in digestion and balance of blood sugar.

Soybean Dish

   4 oz. soybeans

   2 carrots, diced

   2 sprigs parsley

   1 Tbs. hot pressed sesame oil (to taste)

   ½ Tbs. salt

Soak soybeans in water for 2 hours. Clean. Put in pot with enough water to cover. Add salt. Bring to boil, reduce heat, and simmer for ½ hour or until soft. Drain.

Remove leaves on parsley. Remove skins of carrots.

Dip parsley and carrots in boiling water and remove immediately.

Combine carrots and parsley with beans and add sesame oil. Taste. Make adjustments. Serve.

Benefits
This dish reduces blood pressure and cleans the bloodstream. It is detoxifying. It cleans the kidneys and reduces the amount of water in the body.

Eggplant with Mushrooms

  10 oz. eggplant

  10-15 small pieces skin mushroom (black fungus)

  ½ cup vegetable oil

  3 Tbs. vegetable oil

  1 small can water chestnuts, sliced

  1 Tbs. green onion, diced

  1 Tbs. ginger, diced

  1 Tbs. garlic, diced

  ½ red pepper, dried or fresh, diced

  2 Tbs. soy sauce

  1 Tbs. sugar

  2 Tbs. vinegar

  ½ tsp. salt

  2 Tbs. cornstarch mixed in water

  ⅛ tsp. white pepper

  1 tsp. hot pressed sesame oil (to taste)

Clean eggplant, cut in half lengthwise, remove seeds, cut into 1″ cubes.

Soak mushrooms in warm water for 30 minutes. Slice.

In pan, heat ½ cup vegetable oil and fry eggplant for about 5 minutes until they show signs of browning. Drain on paper towel.

In pan, heat 3 Tbs. vegetable oil and over low heat stir fry mushrooms, water chestnuts, green onion, ginger, garlic, and red pepper; be careful not to burn. Combine with eggplant and add soy sauce, sugar, vinegar, and salt. Then add cornstarch. Over medium heat, cover and cook for 5-6 minutes. Garnish with white pepper and sesame oil. Serve.

Benefits
This dish is good for overall detoxification and thyroid function.

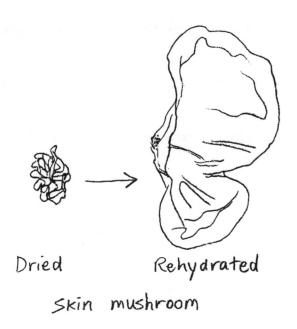

Dried   Rehydrated

Skin mushroom

Tofu Salad

1 package tofu, rinsed and cubed

1 big or 2 small tomatoes

½ tsp. salt

½ Tbs. hot pressed sesame oil

1 Tbs. soy sauce

Soak tomatoes in hot, almost boiling water, for 1 minute. Peel and remove seeds. Dice.

Boil tofu in water for 5 minutes. Drain. Dry and sparingly salt. Drain again.

Add tomato to tofu. Add salt, sesame oil, and soy sauce. Serve.

Benefits
This dish is good for cleansing blood vessels and the brain, and it fights cholesterol.

Cucumber Salad

  1 whole cucumber, peeled, sliced, and rinsed very clean

  4 Tbs. vinegar

  4 Tbs. sugar

  ½ tsp. salt

  1 tsp. soy sauce

  2 Tbs. hot pressed sesame oil

  4 Tbs. water

Slice cucumber lengthwise into halves. Bring a pot of water to boil, dip cucumber in water for 1 minute, remove seeds, and drain.

Combine vinegar, sugar, salt, soy sauce, and sesame oil. Pour on cucumber, refrigerate one hour, and serve.

Benefits
This dish is good for cleaning the blood vessels.

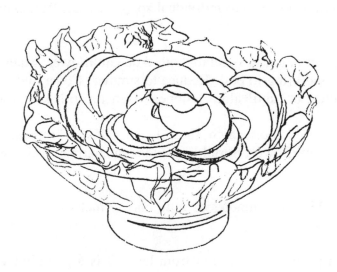

Cauliflower in Milk

1 cauliflower

2 Tbs. vegetable oil

1 green onion, chopped

1 Tbs. water

½ tsp. salt

1 cup milk

1 Tbs. cornstarch

1 Tbs. flour

4 oz. cheddar cheese, shredded

1 Tbs. Parmesan cheese, shredded

½ cup vegetable broth

¼ tsp. salt

¼ cup vegetable broth

Separate cauliflower into individual sprigs. Clean. Peel skin off of stalks.

Sautee green onion in vegetable oil. Add cauliflower, water, and ½ tsp. salt, and bring to boil. Reduce to simmer. Cover and cook for 3-5 minutes, or until almost done. Transfer to baking tray.

In pan, heat milk, cornstarch, flour, ¼ tsp. salt, and broth until thick. Pour over cauliflower. Sprinkle cheddar and parmesan cheeses over dish.

Bake at 325° for 5 minutes or until cheese melts.

Benefits
This dish provides protection from heat. It is a good hot weather food.

180

Asparagus in Milk

1 lb. asparagus, cleaned and white stalk removed

½ cup vegetable broth

2 tsp. salt

1 cup milk

2 Tbs. flour

2 Tbs. vegetable oil

1 tomato

Put 6 cups of water into pot and bring to boil. Add asparagus and boil for 2 minutes. Drain and transfer to plates.

Combine broth, salt, and flour in milk.

In pan, heat vegetable oil and add milk mixture. Bring to boil while constantly stirring until thick, and pour over asparagus.

Soak tomato in hot, almost boiling, water for 1 minute. Peel, dice, add to asparagus and serve.

Benefits
This dish soothes the lungs, reduces mucus, decongests, and reduces water retention.

Silver and Gold Mushrooms

PART I

   8 dried Chinese mushrooms (Tentius edodes)

   1 Tbs. vegetable oil

   ½ tsp. ginger, minced

   1 small can bamboo shoots, sliced

   2 Tbs. soy sauce

   ½ tsp. wine

   salt to taste

   ½ cup vegetable broth

   1 Tbs. cornstarch mixed with a little water

Soak dried mushrooms in water, discard stem, and quarter each one.

In pan, heat vegetable oil, sautee ginger, bamboo shoots, and Chinese mushrooms. Add 1 Tbs. soy sauce, wine, and vegetable broth, and cook 3 minutes. Add cornstarch and rest of soy sauce. Add salt. Set on one side of plate.

PART II

   2 Tbs. vegetable oil

   ½-1 tsp. ginger, minced

   4 oz. fresh mushrooms

   2 oz. water chestnuts

   salt to taste

   ½ tsp. wine

½ cup vegetable broth

1 Tbs. cornstarch mixed with a little water

Clean mushrooms. In pan, heat vegetable oil and add ginger, mushrooms, water chestnuts, salt, wine, and broth. Cook 1 minute. Add 1 Tbs. cornstarch and cook until thick. Place on other side of plate.

Garnish with 1 tsp. hot pressed sesame oil and ⅛ tsp. pepper and serve.

Benefits
This dish is an overall body builder and cancer fighter. It also beautifies.

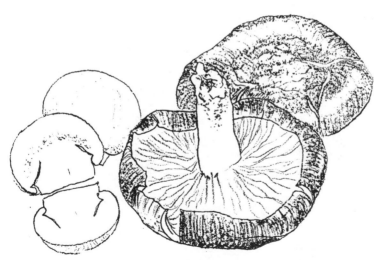

Chinese mushrooms

Plain Rice

2 cups rice (white), uncooked

water to cover rice 1″

Clean rice in pot by rinsing 3-4 times and churning with hand. (Most chemicals will be removed, including the whitener.) Drain.

Add water to rice. Cover. Bring to boil. Reduce to simmer and cook for 30 minutes, stirring occasionally.

Benefits
Steamed rice is a neutral food. It can balance all dishes. It is naturally acid and alkaline balanced. White rice is recommended since brown rice is indigestible because of the shell.

Rice Soup

1 cup rice (white), uncooked

5 cups water

Wash rice, add water, and bring to boil. Reduce to low heat and cook for 1 hour.

Combine with any dish and serve.

Benefits
Rice soup soothes the internal organs. It is good for people who have weak stomachs. It is also good for indigestion, fermentation, and extreme fatigue. It aids in absorption. It can be combined with any dish to soothe and relax the body.

DESSERTS

Peaches with Almonds

4 peach halves

⅓ tsp. lemon rind, grated

4 Tbs. honey

1½ Tbs. lemon juice

½ cup almonds, slivered

1 cup water

¼ tsp. cinnamon

Place peach halves open side up in casserole dish.

combine lemon rind, honey, lemon juice, almonds, and water.

Cover peach halves with mixture. Sprinkle with cinnamon.

Bake for 30 minutes at 325° F. Serve hot or cold.

Orange Pudding

1 package unflavored gelatin (3 oz.)

1½ cup hot water

2 whole oranges

juice of 1 lemon

¼ cup raw sugar

pinch salt

¼ cup powdered skim milk

¼ cup cold water

¼ tsp. vanilla extract

Clean (brush) 1 orange very well, being sure to remove wax on skin. With a grater, grate only the thin orange-colored layer of skin. Set aside.

Slice orange and squeeze out juice. Combine grated peel and juice. Set aside. Peel other orange. Remove skin from orange slices. Keep orange pulp only. Refrigerate.

Combine gelatin and hot water, add sugar and salt. Then add 1 Tbs. lemon juice. Add orange peel and juice. When cool, pour over orange slices and refrigerate till solid. Combine powdered milk and cold water. Whip until thick and creamy, and add vanilla and ½ tsp. lemon juice. Continue whipping. Pour over gelatin mixture. Refrigerate again. Garnish with grated orange skin, slice into cubes, and serve.

Banana Cream Pudding

   5 Tbs. powdered skim milk

   2½ Tbs. flour

   2½ cups water

   2½ Tbs. raw sugar

   2½ lb. bananas, blended until creamy

Combine powdered milk and flour with 2 Tbs. water. Blend until creamy.

Pour rest of water into small pot, bring to boil. Add milk/flour mixture, and add sugar and banana.

Cool and refrigerate, then serve.

Almond Pudding

   2 packages unflavored gelatin

   3½ cups hot water

   10 Tbs. powdered skim milk

   2 tsp. almond extract

   ⅓ cup raw sugar

   ½ cup roasted almonds, finely chopped

   1 cup melted chocolate (optional)

Melt gelatin in hot water and add powdered milk, almond extract, and sugar. Cool. Refrigerate. Sprinkle with roasted almonds and melted chocolate (optional) and serve.

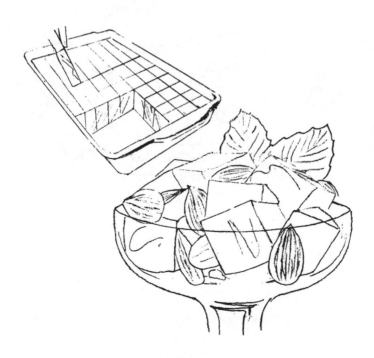

Bean Pudding

½ lb. red beans (from Oriental food store)

2 packages unflavored gelatin

¾ cup raw sugar

5 cups water

pinch salt

Put water in pot, add beans, sugar, and salt. Bring to boil, then reduce to simmer. Cook for at least 4 hours. When almost done, add gelatin. Cool. Refrigerate.

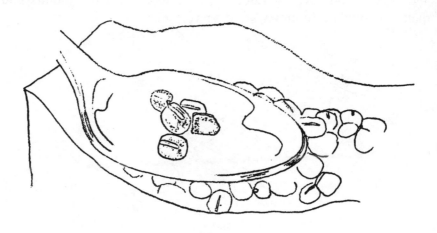

Silver Skin Mushroom Soup

4 oz. silver skin mushroom (from Chinese grocery store)

2 cups water

2 Tbs. raw sugar

1 tsp. almond or cinnamon extract

Place mushrooms in a bowl with enough warm water to cover. Soak for 5 minutes, then clean very well.

Place water and sugar in pan. Bring to boil and add mushrooms.

Reduce to simmer to cook for 5 minutes.

Add almond or cinnamon extract and serve.

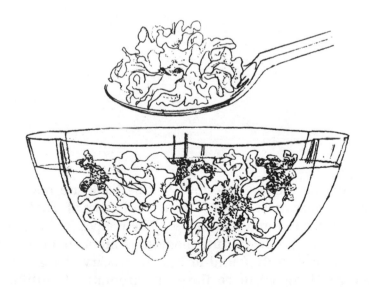

Apple Honey Tea

4 cups apple juice

1 tsp. honey

1 stick cinnamon

4 whole cloves

2 black tea bags or Lipton tea bags

rum (optional)

Combine apple juice, honey, cinnamon, and cloves in pot. Bring to boil.

Remove from heat. Add tea bags, cover, and let sit 10 minutes.

Add rum (optional). Serve with any cake or nuts.

Most of the recipes described in this book are not Chinese recipes, because most Chinese dishes fall short of Taoist standards, though a few may come close. The recipes in this book are Taoist recipes for healthful, modern, American meals. Most ingredients are easily found at nearby grocery stores. And the recipes are designed to be flavorful, aromatic, beautiful, and healthful, while being easy to prepare and economical with time and money.

8

Weight Loss
Testimonials

Jana B.:

In my later teen years I began putting on more and more weight. I felt too heavy and bloated all the time. I was very negative toward my body and I was searching for ways to become thin.

I tried diet after diet. I went on the U.S. Ski Team diet, the Stewardess diet, Dr. Atkins', the Scarsdale, plus many more bizarre patterns of eating and at times I went to the extreme of no food intake at all. I drank diet sodas, ate diet bread, and put diet dressing on my salad. It was a constant battle! Depression and failure became a way of life for me. At times my weight would drop, but I would look sick and feel weak, and in days the weight would be back on.

My preoccupation with food and weight began to run my life. After almost five years of torturing my body I was introduced to Dr. Chang's principles of food and diet. My body was weak but the plan began to strengthen me. I started feeling so much better. No more than a year ago I made the decision to put trust in the food principles of Dr. Chang. I began faithfully eating three meals a day, taking herbs, and lowering my fluid intake. Soon the extra weight was coming off. I have now lost over fifteen pounds and feelings of deprivation and failure no longer control me. I am stronger both physically and emotionally.

Mr. Derudder:

This is my medical history: last year I had a heart attack and had bypass surgery, yet my cholesterol level still remains high at 280 pt. I lived in fear of another heart attack. Then a friend of mine introduced Dr. Chang's weight loss method. After getting on the diet and exercise program, the chest pain and pressure, dry coughs, and irregular heart beats completely disappeared. I can't wait to tell everybody about this.

Ann H.:

I used to weigh 240 pounds. Whenever I looked in the mirror I was tempted to commit suicide. One day I heard about [Dr. Chang's] weight loss method. That method included a way to remove cellulite, and I thought it was exceptional in that it offered a way to remove cellulite permanently. So I religiously followed [Dr. Chang's] instructions. And in three months I was down to 160 pounds. I know I still have a few more pounds of water to eliminate, but I'm still working on it. Thank you.

John Lindseth, Ph.D.:

In my role as an herbologist, I frequently deal with the problems of diet and weight control. In recommending the use of the Internal Exercises, herbs, and other elements of Taoist healing techniques for my clients and then observing the results, I have come to see clearly the enormous value of these techniques for our daily health and well-being. For those who will apply even moderate diligence in the use of the principles outlined in this book, the results are nothing short of miraculous. And even more astonishing to me is that the improvements in health attained by people are lasting. The loss of weight can be permanent, and the efforts are not entirely lost if a person should "forget" to practice the principles for a few days or weeks. To me this is an important test as to the efficacy of the methods employed. They truly do bring lasting improvement.

One instance that comes to mind is the case of a 19 year old girl who within about a six month period lost enough weight to reduce her dress size from 11/12 to 6/7. She did this by eating three meals a day and doing all the things normal to a girl of that age *except* she did them in accordance with the principles of this book. This to me is such an important point. She did not have to dramatically alter her lifestyle to attain drastically better health and her *ideal* weight. It was simply the natural result of using these principles and methods in daily life.

One thing in particular that has struck me is that some of these ideas are so deceptively simple and direct that in very little time whoever practices these methods can quickly experience dramatic benefits. One example of this phenomenon is with people who are overweight largely from retained water. The idea that excessive water is responsible for their overweight condition seems so simple that even when they demonstrate that reducing their water intake reduces their weight, they can hardly believe it. It must, it seems, be more complicated than this—but often it is not. This new (to us) premise that excessive liquid consumption results in retained water and excessive weight will, I believe, be one of the great contributions of our time to the legions of weight watchers.

Other overweight conditions are more complicated, of course, but in any case Dr. Chang has given us the data and tools to understand all of the causes of over- or underweight conditions. He has provided a simple diet plan with numerous recipes so that people can immediately begin to improve their health and at the same time lower their weight. We have both the theoretical data to understand the ''whys''—and the practical tools to prove to ourselves the soundness of the theory—by losing as much weight as we wish.

Recently an article appeared in the newspapers depicting the battle between two leading proponents of well-known diet plans. Each represents a plan which in its details is almost the opposite of the other. Each plan points to the weakness of the other plan and gives detailed information as to the symptoms and illnesses it will cause.

Whichever plan we chose, even if we lose weight, it would be at the expense of our overall health. What a confusing choice to have to make!

Now the most recent popular diet proposes that it makes no difference what a person eats so long as they eat it in a certain order. So we have three well-known plans, and three conflicting theories.

What a relief to have data which we all intuitively know to be sound. It *does* matter what we eat. We *do* need all kinds of food. Extremes of diet *are* likely to be harmful to our health. If our bodies are weakened, our goal of ideal weight *will* be all the harder to attain.

The principles of Taoist weight control have the advantage of being tested and refined for *thousands* of years. Finally we have a *complete* approach to understanding what to eat in order to insure balanced health and a long life at our *ideal* weight.

In my role as a psychotherapist I encourage people to use herbal supplements as an adjunct to their normal diet. This practice has enabled me to see very distinctly the connection between physical health and mental well-being. Often it seems like a few months of herbal supplements will result in improvements in the mental and emotional states of people that experience has shown normally takes many months longer when using a purely psychological approach. Of course the principles of Taoism have for thousands of years taught that weakness or imbalance of certain internal organs will result in a corresponding emotional or mental imbalance. Now after watching this phenomenon occur many, many times I am completely convinced of the validity of this connection between body and mind. Physical well-being means mental and emotional well-being, and vice-versa. Thus on the basis of mind *and* body I can without reservation recommend the principles and methods Dr. Chang has given us in this book.

Index

197

198

Index